# MOTHERING AGAINST THE ODDS

# Mothering Against the Odds

## DIVERSE VOICES
## OF CONTEMPORARY MOTHERS

*Edited by*

CYNTHIA GARCÍA COLL
JANET L. SURREY
KATHY WEINGARTEN

THE GUILFORD PRESS
New York   London

© 1998 The Guilford Press
A Division of Guilford Publications, Inc.
72 Spring Street, New York, NY 10012

Printed in the United States of America

This book is printed on acid-free paper.

Last digit is print number:  9  8  7  6  5  4  3  2  1

**Library of Congress Cataloging-in-Publication Data**

Mothering against the odds : diverse voices of contemporary
    mothers / edited by Cynthia García Coll, Janet L. Surrey, Kathy
    Weingarten.
        p.  cm.
    Includes bibliographical references and index.
    ISBN 1-57230-330-1. — ISBN 1-57230-339-5 (pbk.)
    1. Mothers.  2. Motherhood.  3. Problem families.    I.
García Coll, Cynthia T.  II. Surrey, Janet L.  III. Weingarten,
Kathy.
HQ759.M878   1998
306.874'3—dc21                                        97-47699
                                                          CIP

*For all mothers whose voices are still not heard*

# Contributors

LAURA BENKOV, PhD, is a clinical psychologist in private practice in Brookline, Massachusetts. She received her PhD from City University of New York and is currently an instructor in psychiatry at Harvard Medical School and a supervisor at Children's Hospital, Boston. She is the author of *Reinventing the Family: The Emerging Story of Lesbian and Gay Parents,* published by Crown Publishers in 1994. She is also the mother of a daughter and son.

PHYLLIS BUCCIO-NOTARO, BA, is the executive director of Social Justice for Women (SJW), in Boston, Massachusetts, and oversees the day-to-day operations of six programs targeted to serve women in conflict with the law. Previous to this position, she served as associate director of SJW. She has over 20 years experience working for many leading nonprofit agencies serving women. Ms. Buccio-Notaro has a BA degree from Suffolk University in Boston, and she is currently a candidate for a MA in Criminal Justice, also at Suffolk. In addition, she has been a presenter at many national forums, including the American Society for Criminology, the Academy of Criminal Justice Sciences, and the Center for Substance Abuse Treatment.

PATRICIA FLANAGAN, MD, is a pediatrician and the director of the Teens with Tots Program at Hasboro Children's Hospital in Providence, Rhode Island. In her medical practice, she has specialized in caring for the children of teen mothers for the last 5 years. She is an assistant professor of pediatrics at Brown University. She has three children.

MARILYN G. FRAKTMAN, RN, PhD, has been practicing clinical nursing for over 30 years. Over the past years of her nursing career, she has focused on health-related issues of children, parents, and families. Presently she is a home-visiting nurse for new mothers, babies, and young children. She has recently completed her doctoral dissertation, which emphasizes the need for postpartum support, especially for first-time parents. She is the mother of three adult children.

CYNTHIA GARCÍA COLL, PhD, is a native-born Puerto Rican who has spent half of her life in the northeastearn United States. She is the mother of three children, who are being raised in a multicultural family. Professionally, she is professor of education, psychology, and pediatrics at Brown University, where she teaches and conducts research, and is former director of the Stone Center, Wellesley College, Wellesley, Massachusetts.

MIRIAM GREENSPAN, MEd, LMHC, a pioneer of the feminist therapy movement and author of *A New Approach to Women and Therapy* (McGraw/Hill, 1993), has been a therapist in private practice, writer, consultant, workshop facilitator and public speaker for 25 years. Her essays on feminist psychology and psychotherapy have appeared in *Common Boundary, Ms.,* the journal *Women and Therapy,* and other magazines and anthologies. She lives in Boston with her husband and two daughters, aged 12 and 15.

REBECCA KOCH, MA, LMHC, is a psychotherapist, educator, and consultant. Among the several programs that she has developed for women over the past 20 years, she began and for 5 years directed Cape Ann Families, a family support center sponsored by Wellspring House, Inc., in Gloucester, Massachusetts. She is currently in private practice in Gloucester, specializing in women's issues. She is the mother of a school-age daughter.

MARY T. LEWIS, LICSW, has been a social worker since 1972, working with families. She has worked and lectured both in Asia and within the United States. She is presently working at Wellspring House, Inc., in Gloucester, Massachusetts, and with Cape Ann Families. She is also the mother of four sons, aged 14 to 29.

BARBARA MOLLA, MA, is the clinical director of Social Justice for Women (SJW), in Boston, Massachusetts. In this position, she oversees the clinical continuity of the six criminal justice programs administered by SJW. Ms. Molla has been with SJW for 8 years; immediately prior to her appointment as clinical director, she had served as treatment supervisor at the Neil J. Houston House in Boston, a nationally recognized model of residential service to pregnant women involved with the criminal justice system. Ms. Molla has a long history of work in the fields of substance abuse and women's issues, including service to women in conflict with the law, both with SJW and Women, Inc., a pioneer organization in working with women and their children, also in Boston.

BONNIE Y. OHYE, PhD, is a third-generation Japanese American psychologist, reared and educated in California, now raising her own biracial, bicultural daughters in their home near Boston. She is clinical instructor in psychology at Harvard Medical School, where she teaches and supervises psychologists and psychiatrists in training. She is also a member of the board of directors of the Massachusetts Psychological Association.

WENDY QUIÑONES, M.A., one of four daughters, is now the mother of two sons. After nearly 20 years as a journalist, she has for the last 6 years developed and facilitated education programs with women who are homeless, low income, or otherwise in transition. She is associate program coordinator at the Veronese Community Education Resource Center at Wellspring House, Inc., in Gloucester, Massachusetts.

PHOEBE KAZDIN SCHNITZER, PhD, has a long-standing interest in single-parent families, stemming from years of consultation to community daycare and Head Start programs. She has been at the Judge Baker Children's Center, practicing and teaching child and family psychotherapy for more than 25 years, and is also an instructor in the Department of Psychiatry at the Harvard Medical School. Her current writings use a narrative approach to address issues of single mothering, absent fathers, welfare reform, and the impact of poverty on families in therapy. Her son and daughter are both in their 20s.

BETSY SMITH, PhD, is a lesbian mother of two adopted children and has been an activist in progressive social movements for many years. She is a clinical psychologist both in private practice and at Fenway Community Health Center in Boston. In her practice she has written about, spoken about, and worked extensively with gay and lesbian families.

ELIZABETH SPARKS, PhD, is an assistant professor in the Counseling, Developmental Psychology, and Research Methods Department at Boston College. She earned her PhD in Counseling Psychology at Boston College in 1988. Her research interests stem from a 17-year clinical career in community mental health and a focus on interpersonal, assaultive violence in African American youth and issues in multicultural counseling and training. She is an African American woman who has worked with children and families for most of her professional career, and she has also been an "other mother" and "auntie" to a number of children.

JANET L. SURREY, PhD, has been committed to studying and facilitating women's development for the past 20 years. She is currently codirector of the Gender Relations Project and founding scholar of the Jean Baker Miller Training Institute at the Stone Center, Wellesley College, Wellesley, Massachusetts; attending psychologist at McLean Hospital, Harvard Medical School; and a clinical psychologist in private practice in Boston. She is the coauthor of *Women's Growth in Connection: Writings from the Stone Center* (Guilford, 1991) and contributor to *Women's Growth in Diversity: More Writings from the Stone Center* (Guilford, 1997). She is also the mother of a 6-year-old daughter adopted from China.

MARY WATKINS, PhD, is committed to finding ways for psychology—through theory creation, psychological praxis, and research—to be a liberatory activity. She is the chair of the Master's Program in Counseling Psychology at Pacifica Graduate Institute in Santa Barbara, California. She is the author of *Waking Dreams* (Harper & Row, 1976) and *Invisible Guests: The Development of Imaginal Dialogues* (Analytic Press, 1986), coauthor of *Talking with Young Children about Adoption* (Yale University Press, 1993), and coeditor of *Psychology and the Promotion of Peace* (special issue, *Journal of Social Issues*). She is the stepmother of three children, and the mother of three daughters, adopted from Brazil, India, and China.

KATHY WEINGARTEN, PhD, has been using first-person narrative to ground clinical theorizing for a decade. She is an assistant professor of psychology at Harvard Medical School, codirector of the Program in

Narrative Therapies at The Family Institute of Cambridge, and a practicing therapist. She is the author of *The Mother's Voice: Strengthening Intimacy in Families* (Guilford, 1997) and author or editor of four other books and numerous articles and chapters. She is the mother of a young-adult son and daughter.

KAREN FRASER WYCHE, PhD, is an assistant professor at the Ehrenkranz School of Social Work of New York University. She is a fellow of the American Psychological Association, Division of the Psychology of Women (Div. 35) and was a Bunting Institute Fellow at Radcliffe College. Her research interests include social supports in minority women and gender and ethnic understanding in children.

# Acknowledgments

No book emerges without a history and without support. We thank the original members of the study group on mothers—Laura Benkov, Marilyn G. Fraktman, Kathy Kendall-Tackett, Sally Mack, Chris Robb, Betsy Smith, and Mary Watkins—for engaging with us in those early conversations before we had found our way.

Two women in our community were instrumental in transforming our study group on mothers into a work group to write a book about mothers. In 1994, Dr. Jessica Henderson Daniel organized a conference "Mothers: Faces and Phases." Dr. Daniel's enthusiasm for the topic and her rigorous intellectual formulation of the issue of diversity in relation to mothers encouraged us in our work and set a standard we wanted to meet.

Later, we approached Barbara Watkins, now our editor for this book, to see whether or not she might be interested in publishing our work. True to the spirit of collaboration on this project and her own intellectual integrity, she not only agreed to shepherd the project through the publication process but also to come to our meetings and work with us in shaping the structure and themes of the book. She has read every chapter once, some many times, and has given us invaluable editorial assistance even before the manuscript formally crossed her desk.

Each of the contributors to this book has attended monthly meetings to discuss the chapters written by other contributors. These conversations have been vital to the shaping of each author's work. We are grateful to all of them for their generosity in reading and critiquing each other's papers and for the lively discussions that led to the three conversations.

At the time that the group met at the Stone Center for Developmental Services and Studies at Wellesley College, from 1993 to 1995, Mary Melo was instrumental in handling the logistics of our meetings. In 1995–1996, Katherine Magnuson ably assisted the book's progress and in 1996–1997, Suzie Nacar took over the task. Suzie's good humor is matched by her thoughtfulness and precision. She has been unflagging in her efforts on the book's behalf—calling, typing, e-mailing, and faxing—in short, meticulously doing whatever we needed done.

We were fortunate to have Kate O'Shea transcribe the conversations. She also did a remarkable analysis of the themes of the first meeting's discussion.

Kathy Weingarten's 89-year-old mother-in-law, Eleanor Goddard Worthen, copyedited each of the chapters. Her meticulous, thoughtful reading and her unswerving interest in this project has been an inspiration and a boon to us.

Finally, the Education Department at Brown University provided many in-kind contributions that made the book possible.

I, Cynthia, would like to thank my children, Nat, Andrés, and Gabriela, for their patience and tolerance at not being put to bed by me so many Wednesday nights when I was in Boston.

I, Jan, thank my family for hosting our whole group for our monthly meetings in our living room. I am especially grateful to my daughter, Katie, and my mother, Rosalie, for inspiring me to do this work.

I, Kathy, would also like to thank my daughter, Miranda Eve Weingarten Worthen, who graciously accepted the three of us sprawling in the kitchen every other Wednesday afternoon for 2 years.

We three have had a wonderful time working together. Perhaps the clearest indication of our pleasure in the collaboration is that we are hatching plans for our next project. The three of us have contributed equally to the creation of this book and we have chosen to list our names alphabetically.

CYNTHIA GARCÍA COLL
JANET L. SURREY
KATHY WEINGARTEN

*Preface*

History, especially women's history, can be written on many levels. This book came into being through the creative interchange of many of the book's contributors as part of a study group on mothers' psychological development at the Stone Center at Wellesley College. We are a diverse group of women and mothers by age, sexuality, culture, race, class, religious background, age of children, and biological/adoptive status, among others. We represent many, but clearly not all, of the different contexts of mothering. We are also a group of professionals—clinicians, researchers, educators, theoreticians, and writers—all committed to studying and supporting families. In this book we focus on mothers, especially those whose mothering practices or contexts have been marginalized. But we are equally committed to the support of fathers who also struggle to care for families. Indeed, although this book does not challenge the many constraining ideas about fathers and fathering, we vigorously support those professionals who have taken up this task (Levant, 1995; Osherson, 1986; Pleck, 1985; Pruett, 1987; Silverstein & Rashbaum, 1994).

This book developed from our concern that the voices of mothers, speaking of their (our) own subjective experiences, are not being heard or well represented in the mainstream cultural discourses of psychological development, clinical practice, or social policy. We are also concerned that the diverse, often difficult, contexts shaping mothers' experiences are often invisible, and that the unique strengths of mothers within these contexts are often unrecognized. We believe that mother blaming continues, despite three decades of work identifying its pernicious effects and the false premises latent therein (Caplan, 1989; Thurer, 1994).

Clinicians and researchers, as well as politicians and social commentators, still blame mothers for their children's problems and also for larger societal problems. We are all too aware that mothers tend to internalize this pervasive, immense sense of responsibility and blame.

We wanted to find ways to articulate and construct our own "personal" experiences as women and mothers as part of, and not apart from, our "professional" life and work commitments. Perhaps most importantly, we sought other "mother/professionals" with whom we could develop new perceptions, new constructions, and new understandings of the forces that shape mothers' experience in different contexts. What brought us together was the intuitive sense that something of value would come from connecting with each other. We each had a sense that our own personal and intellectual isolation and our marginalization as mothers expressed a deep truth about mothers. Our lived reality seemed missing from the dominant ideologies reflected in current "expert knowledge." Many of us had the sense that the richness, complexity, and power of our own and other mothers' experience had not been fully brought forth and that we needed to create community for this to happen.

At a very personal level, the impetus for convening the group came from Jan Surrey's adoption of her daughter, Katie Chun, from China, in March 1992. First-time motherhood, the impact of adoption, and the power of cross-racial mothering led to a powerful yearning for connection and community to help construct meaning for these experiences, to find avenues for building on such meanings, and for creating opportunities for other marginalized mothers' voices to be "heard into speech" (Morton, 1985).

I, Jan, began talking with significant "mother" friends and mentors about creating such a study group, which first met in the fall of 1993. As a researcher, clinician, and theoretician at the Stone Center, I sought out a number of women who were already central figures in my mothering network. Mary Watkins, clinician, educator, and writer, had been a particular "mother–mentor" for me, as the mother of three internationally adopted daughters and as a former colleague in a group seeking to articulate global frameworks for psychotherapy.

Cynthia García Coll was director of the Stone Center (1991–1994) at that time and had, just before Katie's arrival, loaned me the crib she had used for her three children, which her youngest child had just outgrown. She also gave me my copy of Penelope Leach's *Your Baby and Child* (1990). Cynthia and I were beginning to work together on the Stone Center mission integrating cultural diversity into the core of the work of the Center. As director, she was instrumental in supporting the early work of this group.

Sometime after returning from China, I received a welcome home note from Kathy Weingarten, whom I had never actually met. She sent some of her early writing on mothers and an invitation to call on her daughter, then 13, for baby-sitting, as she lived close by. I remember Kathy's papers sitting on my floor unread for many months during that period of early mothering when I read nothing. Yet it was an invitation to connection that would later lead me to invite her to the first meeting of this group at the Stone Center. Since then, each of us has invited others to join; some have come and gone.

This book was born from conversation and colleagueship, argument and awareness. In 1993, when Jan and Cynthia convened the group for the first time at the Stone Center, we were a group of eight with disparate professional backgrounds and a converging interest in mothers. As academics, researchers, clinicians, and mothers, many of us wore several hats.

The first and second years were ones of finding common ground that would allow us to pursue with enough depth and clarity the material we were engaged in studying. Eventually, slowly, and with deliberate effort, we found concepts that allowed us to organize our agreements and disagreements. Initially the concepts of risk, resilience, and resistance were the ones that provided a meeting place, a location in which our different points of view overlapped sufficiently so that we could hear and respond to each other's work with insight and rigor.

These conversations were stimulating and thought provoking. As the membership of the group changed, retaining a stable core, the openings in the group provided opportunities to include the voices and perspectives of mothers in various contexts of resistance. As we developed a vocabulary to talk fluently with each other, we developed the idea of creating a book to share this experience with others.

In putting together the frameworks for this book, we knew we wanted to hear the voices of a diverse group of mothers but we also wanted to recognize commonalities among them. Marginalization and resistance captured for us our twin interests. In order to give the chapters some internal consistency, we developed guidelines for chapter contributors, through a collaborative process of conversation stretched over several meetings. The guidelines posed questions and gave examples of topics that we felt mapped the territory in relation to mothers, marginalization, and resistance.

The process of selecting contributors who had not already been study group members followed the logic of the group's process. Besides the criterion of working with mothers from a marginalized group, or mothers whose mothering practices diverged from the Eurocentric "norm," we wanted to include women who might be able to participate in our monthly meetings. We wanted as much as possible for the chapters to be influenced by dialogue about each other's work. When this was not possible, we invited women with whom we had had collegial relationships in other contexts, women with whom we had already been in dialogue. In this way, we created what we might call an opportunistic sample. Or, put another way, we were creating one of many such possible communities of voices: communities of diverse maternal stories.

Editing the book fell to Jan, Cynthia, and Kathy, three members of the original study group, and the three who had maintained momentum about the project most consistently through the years. In collaboration with other members of the study group, our book proposal was accepted by The Guilford Press in the spring of 1996, at the end of the third year of our meeting together.

## SITUATING OUR OWN PERSONAL AND PROFESSIONAL CONTEXTS

The three of us share an understanding of the importance of acknowledging the relevance of our personal lives and social locations in shaping our passions, life commitments, and professional values and directions. For this reason, we are including brief biographical statements that situate this work in the context of our personal and professional lives.

For me, Jan, my own coming of age was shaped by the 1960s and the women's liberation movement, which sought to reconstruct the ideologies of "womanhood" within the social and historical context of late 20th-century capitalist patriarchy. My feminism as well as my theoretical work articulating a relational model of women's psychological development were part of my lifelong attempts to understand and negotiate the paradoxes within my relationship with my mother. I spent many years in therapy being instructed to blame, pathologize, and "separate" from my mother. This strategy never worked for me, as I have always been deeply connected and enormously inspired as well as wounded and confused in this relationship.

My description of the healthy desire for and obstacles to connection in the mother–daughter relationship has been shaped by my relationship. I have been writing about and walking my way out of mother blaming for the past 20 years, and I am still passionately committed to honoring and supporting the potentially positive power of mother–daughter relationships.

Six years ago, in 1991, I traveled to China to adopt my daughter, Katie, who has become the light and joy of my life. Mothering in this context has opened me up to whole new aspects of mothering: international and interracial adoption, midlife mothering, and, most powerfully, living as a family of color in this culture. These are the contexts, I suspect, that will shape my further explorations of mothering, both personally and now professionally.

I, Cynthia, am a native-born Puerto Rican woman who migrated to the continental United States at the age of 22 to pursue graduate education. I have now lived here for over 20 years. I grew up in an atypical (mother, grandmother, and daughter), middle-class family in a suburb of San Juan, and because of that upbringing I have always been an observer of human nature. I also saw my mother's struggles as a single mother, the many pressures laid upon her, and the consequences these circumstances had upon us.

My first research with mothers was conducted in Puerto Rico in 1976. This marked the beginning of my interest in teenage mothers and their experience (and that of their children), as well as my interest in the influence of the dominant culture on their immediate circumstances. Studies that I have conducted with other atypical populations such as children with high-risk medical conditions at birth, major developmental difficulties, or atypical temperaments have also made me aware of the many challenges that mothers face and that society tends to dismiss or negate. The extent of mothers' self-sacrifices and their ability to cope with everything—from breastfeeding a 2-pound newborn to raising a child who is disabled or has a difficult temperament—is astonishing. However, just as astonishing is society's inability or unwillingness to recognize the true difficulty of all of these endeavors.

I also bring to this book my own personal experience as a mother of three children in a dual-career, bicultural family. I have become keenly aware through my work and my own experience as a daughter and a mother of how ideologically charged the definition of a "good mother" is in our society.

I, Kathy, have been interested in mothers' lives, in mothers' stories, for as long as I can remember. I found my mother fascinating and she found her mother and mother-in-law so as well. Some of my happiest memories are around small tables in cramped apartment kitchens listening to the tales my immigrant grandmothers told, as my mother elicited them, about their daily lives, mothering in infelicitous circumstances and doing it with élan.

It does not surprise me that my intellectual history is one in which attending to maternal voice is central. Much of my professional career has been an effort to fairly name what mothers do. This effort has been one of storying and re-stor(y)ing. My own life, as a mother and as the daughter of a mother, has been one of the lives with which I have worked (Weingarten, 1995, 1997).

Frequently, questions and experiences in my life have catalyzed my professional inquiry. I have done research on two-career couples and the impact of the timing of parenthood in adult lives. Since 1989, my principal theoretical and clinical focus has been on the application of postmodern thinking to the study of mothers' lives. I have used voice and its silencing as an organizing metaphor. I have been concerned with the contexts in which mothers are listened to well and poorly, and I have tried to identify the mechanisms by which social acts of silencing are transformed into individual experiences of voicelessness. This project opens my vista to a wider range of maternal experience than I have hitherto explored and for this I am grateful.

CYNTHIA GARCÍA COLL
JANET L. SURREY
KATHY WEINGARTEN

## REFERENCES

Caplan, P. (1989). *Don't blame mother: Mending the mother–daughter relationship.* New York: HarperCollins.

Levant, R., with Kopecky, G. (1995). *Masculinity reconstructed: Changing the rules of manhood—At work, in relationships, and in family life.* New York: Dutton.

Leach, P. (1990). *Your baby and child: From birth to age six.* New York: Knopf.

Morton, N. (1985). *The journey is home.* Boston: Beacon Press.

Osherson, S. (1986). *Finding our fathers: The unfinished business of manhood.* New York: Free Press.

Pleck, J. (1995). *Working wives/working husbands.* Newbury Park, CA: Sage.

Pruett, K. D. (1987). *The nurturing father.* New York: Warner Books.

Silverstein, O., & Rashbaum, B. (1994). *The courage to raise good men*. New York: Viking.

Thurer, S. (1994). *The myths of motherhood: How culture reinvents the good mother.* New York: Houghton Mifflin.

Weingarten, K. (Ed.). (1995). *Cultural resistance: Challenging beliefs about men, women, and therapy.* New York: Haworth Press.

Weingarten, K. (1997). *The mother's voice: Strengthening intimacy in families.* New York: Guilford Press. (Originally published 1994 by Harcourt Brace)

# Contents

# Introduction

KATHY WEINGARTEN

JANET L. SURREY

CYNTHIA GARCÍA COLL

MARY WATKINS[1]

FOR most mothers it is impossible to escape the ubiquitous idea that some mothers are "good," others "bad," and that some mothering practices are "right" and others "wrong." These ideas about mothers pervade our lives. Texts, images, interpersonal interactions, codes, and laws all drench us in messages about what constitutes good and bad mothering and who the good and the bad mothers are.

Though this coding of maternal behavior may seem invariant, what we code and how we code it has shifted dramatically over time. The feminist philosopher Elizabeth Badinter concluded that mothers behave as the culture dictates (Badinter, 1981). In her fascinating study of mothering practices in urban France from the 17th to the 20th centuries, Badinter has been able to determine that, for example, in 18th-century urban France, women of all classes did not organize their lives around the care of children, but rather around their husbands' lives. A "good" mother did not breastfeed her children, as she might today, for this would have interfered with her wifely role.

---

[1]Mary Watkins contributed to the writing of the Introduction but was not involved in the editing of the book that this chapter addresses.

If we look at the structure of maternal coding, we can see that dichotomization is its essential feature. Mothers and their behavior are coded as either good or bad. Nancy Chodorow, a psychoanalytically trained sociologist, and Susan Contratto, a psychologist, believe that it is the child's perspective of the mother that the culture has encoded in this dichotomy (Chodorow & Contratto, 1982). The child's fantasy of the perfect mother generates the good–bad split; it also obscures the mother's point of view.

Clinical and developmental psychology have historically focused on child development, with little attention paid to the lifelong relational development of mothers and children; even less attention is paid to the psychological development of mothers. The absence of the mother's perspective and experience in clinical formulations, developmental theory, and psychological research is striking.

The dominant Western ideologies of development portray the evolution of the individual "self" as emerging out of childlike dependence and enmeshment. Mothers are seen as "supports," "matrices," "holding environments," or "self-objects" who supply, gratify, mirror, and "develop" children. Without a two-person or relational psychology of human development, women and mothers will continue to be regarded primarily as "objects" or "self-objects," and not as "subjects" or "selves." In such a paradigm, mothers appearing as subjects with voices and interests of their own are experienced as deeply suspect and potentially destructive to children's development.

For women, the path to adulthood and motherhood remains complicated by the inherent conflict (as culturally constructed) between self-development and relational connection (Braverman, 1989; Surrey, 1990, 1996; Weingarten, 1997). Gilligan, Rogers, and Tolman (1991) have suggested that this core paradox begins to impact young women at adolescence. Surrey (1990, 1996) postulates that this relational paradox is at the core of mothers' lives; that is, in the name of the mothering relationship, mothers begin to take more and more of their authentic experience out of relationship, thus distorting and disempowering themselves and their relationships. This paradox renders mothers both deeply and passionately engaged in connections with their children, but simultaneously disconnected, disempowered, and isolated as mothers in their internal and relational worlds as well as in their social, political, and vocational worlds. It is the task of this book directly to address mothers' subjectivity. It is a project shared with other feminist scholars (Bell-Scott et al., 1991; Daly & Reddy, 1991; Glenn, Chang, & Forcey, 1994; Knowles & Cole, 1990; Reddy, Roth,

& Sheldon, 1994), and it directly undermines the pervasive practices of mother blaming.

All of the contributors to this book share the belief that mother blaming—and the ubiquitous splitting of mothers and mothering into good and bad, right and wrong, that underlies it—has exerted a powerful and destructive influence on family life. One important study looked at the incidence of mother blaming in major clinical journals in 1970, 1976, and 1982 and noted that mothers were blamed for a total of 72 different kinds of psychopathology (Caplan & Hall-McCorquodale, 1985). The frequency of mother blaming did not vary significantly over the 3 target years. The ratio of mentions of the mother to father was 5:1.

Responding to the pervasiveness and destructiveness of mother blaming by clinicians, Jean Baker Miller suggested that "we declare a five- year moratorium on mother blaming in order to be more creative and thoughtful in our clinical formulations and psychotherapy" (Surrey, 1990, p. 86). Nearly a decade later, the challenge is as fresh and the need as great.

## CHANGING CONTEXTS FOR MOTHERING: CHILDCARE ARRANGEMENTS IN AMERICA

Society's definition of "good" mothering is closely tied to particular childcare arrangements. These arrangements, however, are responsive to social and economic factors, not primarily biological ones. The childcare arrangement that white middle-class Americans take for granted consists of care by married women in a nuclear family of children and parents; these women are largely unassisted and isolated. But anthropological studies (Margolis, 1984, pp. 15–16) show that this arrangement differs from that of 93.9% of the world's population. In a study of 186 societies worldwide, in less than half were mothers the primary caretaker of infants. In fewer than 20% of societies was the mother the primary caretaker after infancy (Margolis, 1984). However, in common with the rest of the world's population past and present, we assume our own methods of childcare are the best and the most natural. In fact, we do so despite much evidence to the contrary.

To gain a deeper understanding of their role in American culture, mothers need to appreciate the historical and cultural forces that have crafted their job description and the psychological burden that issues from it. A brief look at American history can show how novel our present images of "mother" are.

Three centuries ago, although all adult women were expected to marry and bear children, the orbit of their industry was far larger than childcare. In colonial America, mothers did not devote themselves to their children. Instead, the mother was a necessary member of the production team and she could not be spared to care for children, who were not seen as valuable until they too were old enough to contribute to the economic survival of the family and the colony (Block, 1978).

Women were responsible for much of the home industry, that is, the production of clothing, food, and all other household goods, and children were integrated at an early age into the work of the family. Older siblings, apprentices, journeymen (i.e., adolescents "put out" to learn a trade), servants, and extended family often also lived in the household. They contributed to the care of the younger children as the mother worked through her daily list of chores. As the children grew, the boys were trained by the father and men, and the girls by the mother and women of the house. Childhood was at most a period lasting up to age 10, but long before that, by age 5 or 6, each child had an orbit of industry. Childhood was not thought of as a period of leisure, play, or protection as we now envision it. Children were conceived of as miniature adults and treated accordingly. There was little attention paid to developing their personalities, their individuality, or their intelligence (Margolis, 1984, p. 19). What attention was paid was not the province of mothers. According to historian John Demos (1983), in the late 1600s it was fathers, not mothers, who were believed to be the central figures in the child's religious and moral development. Men were thought to be better endowed to reason than women, a characteristic that made it necessary for them to be the rulers over children and mothers. "Carried to and fro by their inordinate affections and lacking the 'compass' of sound reason, women could hardly provide the vigilant supervision that all children needed" (Demos, 1983, p. 162).

With the rise of capitalism and industrialism the former arrangements for childcare were disrupted. The idea of the child began to change radically, and with it the idea of who "mother" should be. Production outside the home increased, as store-bought goods began to be substituted for homemade ones. This lessened the burden on women for household production. By the late 1700s the family had become more nuclear. Servants and apprentices were no longer members, and the father worked outside the home for the larger part of the day. For the first time in American history the home and the workplace became separated (Chodorow, 1978, p. 5). Because the man of the family left the home each day for long periods of time, childcare was left exclusively to the mother. As the practice of putting out children into apprenticeships declined, childhood began to reach into what we now call "adolescence," leaving mothers with both older and younger children to care for exclusively.

For the first time, childhood—and an extended one at that—began to be seen as a distinct period in the life cycle. A literature of advice arose that began to warn how crucial the early years were to the later character of the child. The "discovery" of the child led to the "cult of motherhood." Images of mothers became polarized: Mothers were either saintly, all-nurturing, and self-sacrificing; or cruel, ruthless, and self-centered. Although the image of the saintly mother primarily applied to white women of middle- and upper-class status, women of color and women of lower social class were also affected. This ideal became the dominant discourse of expectations of motherhood and often rendered the experiences of women of color and lower social class inferior by comparison (Collins, 1987; Ehrenreich & English, 1979).

As childcare came to be left to mothers who were increasingly freed from other responsibilities, the psychological significance of mothering became elevated in the writings of the late 19th century. Such literature became increasingly addressed to mothers alone, as duties that had been shared or had been the preserve of fathers gradually came within the province of mothers. The mother in popular literature was depicted as the moral guide for both children and husband. While the husband coped with the evils of power, aggression, and ambition outside the home, the wife and mother was supposed to create a protected environment, a haven in which to bring up her children and to which her husband could return to rest and renew himself. The more mothers were idealized and given power to do good, the greater the potential seemed that they might also misuse that power and go astray, promoting evil and badness, and harming their children and society by their wrong doings in the realm of motherhood.

By the time psychology overtook religion in providing the canon for childrearing, mothers were seen as the exclusive care providers for children. Psychoanalytic theory that focuses on the mother–child dyad would not have been possible before the child's early affective relations had been shrunk down to one person. The mother's personality did indeed become central to the developing child, because the child was left alone with the mother. Psychoanalytic theory, unmindful of its cultural context, did not question this arrangement or its consequences for children and mothers. Rather it took these arrangements as universal and inevitable. It could be argued that one factor in the so-called "breakdown of the American family" is the culmination of this century's impossible ideas about motherhood. Now a mother is assigned full-time work outside the home, while she is expected to perform the bulk of childcare, and to attend minutely (largely unassisted) to the emotional and psychological development of her children (far into adulthood), in communities that have failed to provide education, health care, resources, and safety.

## MARGINALIZATION OF MOTHERS

It is precisely in the context of the unrealistic demands placed on contemporary mothers that marginalization of mothers and their mothering practices takes place. Marginalization is the social phenomenon of being diminished and devalued in comparison to others, or of having one's ideas, feelings, practices, or actions rendered less valid or useful in relation to a dominant ideal. When marginalization occurs, the experience of some is subjugated to the experience of others and rendered less visible and less heard. Those who are marginalized often find that their experiences are represented by others in ways that do not express or reflect them. Value is placed on the experiences of those in the center, and less value, no value, or a negative value is placed on those pushed to the margins.

There are many ways that marginalization of mothers occurs. One way is in relation to other mothers. Those at the center tend to be mothers with economic resources, social and community support, and a view of themselves and mothering that fits the dominant ideology. Mothers who are seriously compromised in their ability to access social resources are blamed, mis-seen, or vilified, such as welfare mothers, mothers in prison, mothers who are homeless, or poor immigrant mothers.

In fact, it is possible to describe the prototypical "good mother." She is likely to be white, married, not working in a job that takes her away "too much" from her parenting responsibilities; she has only one or two children, and they do not have any physical defects or behavioral problems; she conceived her children and is raising them in a heterosexual relationship; and she and her spouse are older than 20 years of age and are of the same ethnic and racial background. The more a mother deviates from this prototype, the more likely that she or her mothering practices will be marginalized. These assumptions marginalize the many mothers who are raising competent children and maintaining adaptive family systems, some in spite of very difficult extenuating circumstances.

Another way that mothers are marginalized is in relation to the ideal of the "good mother." No mother can *always* be a good mother by her own or others' standards, and therefore all mothers are inevitably marginalized by this oppressive ideal. Societal marginalization—the social phenomenon—is experienced individually. All of us are affected, even haunted by the cultural images of "good" and "bad" mothers. Most of the authors in this book wrestle profoundly with popular and professional ideas about resilience that imply that children in any context will develop well, regardless of risk and circumstance, *if* there is sufficient "goodness" or "strength" in their individual mothers. These models place mothers at risk. The current political targeting of single mothers, working mothers, and lesbian mothers does just this.

A third way that marginalization of mothers takes place is through the invisibility or absence of representation of their own particular contexts, practices, or preferences in dominant constructions of mothering. Many mothers find their experience missing in cultural iconography. It seems as if the dominant culture wants to expunge their maternal situation or style from the "record." Adoptive mothers, mothers of adolescents and disabled children, and bicultural mothers are marginalized by their lack of representation in discussions and images of mothers. Marginalization breeds invisibility. However, it can also give rise to resistance.

## FROM MARGIN TO CENTER: ACTS OF RESISTANCE

While the culture can marginalize the realities of mothers in many ways, mothers do not have to accept this. Many find ways to actively resist their marginalization.

Each of the chapters in this volume examines sources of resistance and draws on the voices and strengths of the mothers being represented. We chose, as a group, to focus on the concept of resistance to marginalization, rather than psychological resilience. We felt that the concept of resilience as traditionally used in psychology considered the individual apart from the social context, a view that we found unhelpful and misleading. The scope of "resilience" was too broad, encompassing highly individualistic intrapsychic factors, and could easily fall into blaming individual mothers for "nonresilience." The decision to focus on resistance, not resilience, was itself a form of resistance to the traditional categories of psychological and clinical research, which have profoundly silenced and pathologized mothers.

Chapter contributors draw on a variety of theoretical models of resistance, but we have found our theoretical differences to be compatible at the level of basic assumptions, psychological and sociopolitical applications, and personal commitments. With regard to resistance, we have drawn on the work of Weingarten (1995, 1997); Jordan, Kaplan, Miller, Stiver, and Surrey (1991); García Coll, Cook-Nobles, and Surrey (1995); Gilligan et al. (1991); Robinson and Ward (1991); Freire (1989); hooks (1989); Aptheker (1989); and Stacey (1997).

First, it is important to state that we are using the concept of resistance as it has been articulated in the sociopolitical, not the psychological, domain. Resistance as described within the psychological domain has generally been cast in a negative, destructive light. Aware of this, and wanting to retain the concept of resistance nonetheless, Gilligan, founder of the Harvard Project on Girls and Women, reframes and distinguishes positive or "healthy" resistance from more damaging psychological forms, which create psychological symptoms such as anxiety, depression, dissociation, and immobilization (Gilligan et al., 1991). Gilligan's work has influenced our thinking about resistance from a psychological perspective.

However, this book is more concerned with resistance as it is understood within a sociopolitical perspective. We have drawn on the works of several writers who speak about resistance in this way. bell hooks (1989) writes of the movement from margin to center as an act of self-determination as one becomes one's own subjective center; this is an act of resistance, opposition, and liberation for those who have been at the margins. She defines this process of "speaking out" or "talking back" to dominant objectifying forces as liberatory and radically transforming. We see this book as part of and contributing to a more realistic, appreciative, exploratory, and creative construction of motherhood. As hooks writes, "The struggle to end domination, the individual struggle to move from object to subject, is expressed in the effort to establish the liberatory voice—that way of speaking that is no longer determined by one's status as object. That way of speaking is characterized by resistance. It demands that paradigms shift—that we learn to talk—to listen—to hear in a new way" (1989, p. 15).

The work of several authors is helpful in understanding the processes that persons go through to establish a liberatory voice. Paulo Freire (1989), leader of the literacy movement in Brazil, radical pedagogist, and social activist, argues that learning to read should involve a process of becoming able to decode the cultural and socio-economic circumstances that shape your life and your thinking. He calls the first step in this empowering process "conscientization," a group process that allows one to engage actively with the structures one has previously identified with and been blind to. The process allows people to see through these constructions.

In Freire's (1989) model, an "animator" helps group participants to interrogate their day-to-day experience, their concerns and suffering, exploring the relation between daily life and the cultural dictates that suffuse it. Efforts at change are directed not foremost to the individual level, but to wider cultural change that will, in the end, affect the participants. This change becomes possible through the second step of Freire's method, "annunciation." Once a group knows how to decode the dominant paradigm and its effects, then they can begin to conceive of more just social arrangements.

Freire's Brazilian work has direct application in therapeutic and community-oriented work with mothers, as well as in our conceptualization of mothers' lives. It asks of us that we enlarge our understanding of the sufferings of individual mothers to include the historical and cultural contexts that shape their daily lives. Further, it asks that groups of mothers inquire into their deepest intentions and heartfelt aspirations for their relations with their children, and that they work together to change some of the status-quo-oriented forces that mitigate against creating motherhood in ways that more effectively serve mothers and children.

These ideas fit with ours about resistance and mothering. Weingarten, in her work on "cultural resistance" (1995), discusses another aspect of the process by which persons can identify dominant cultural discourses, critique, and resist them. This, she believes, makes room for voice that is authenticated by communities of listeners. Weingarten has applied this framework in therapeutic contexts and in the family (1995, 1997), especially focusing on maternal voice.

Authors at the Stone Center have focused on creating mutually empathic and mutually empowering relational contexts in therapy and in research that empower, authorize, and support the emergence of different voices. In particular, clinicians and researchers have sought to "hear into speech" the voices of girls and women who have "carried" the disavowed knowledge of the worlds of connection and relationship within the dominant culture (Miller, 1976; Jordan et al., 1991). Such a model of resistance seeks to describe with great detail the qualities and radical impact of such "listening," "being present with," "standing with," and "solidarity with" the client or subject. Surrey (García Coll et al., 1996) has described a key aspect of psychological strength in women as the capacity for healthy resistance and described the power of mutually authentic and mutually empathetic relationships as "resistance-fostering" relationships. In patriarchal culture, women's (especially mothers') resistance to division, isolation, and "silencing" lies in the power of authentic connection.

Frequently, in this volume, marginalized mothers speak of close relationships with other mothers and role models as the source of their ability to resist devaluation or vilification and to maintain a sense of worth and hope. This emphasis on the qualities of the listener and the relational context lead to an emphasis on building or accessing "communities of resistance" (Welch, 1985), which appear to be an important factor in each of the models of resistance we draw on. These communities are often politically and/or spiritually based, and may be the foundation on which a liberation movement can develop. They frequently are a source of alternative culture building, through the development of new language, literature, art, music, ritual, and storytelling, and community action, through enlarged communication possibilities through newspapers, workshops and conferences, media alerts, marches, and so forth. Such communities foster the process of resistance and the creation or liberation of new voices and visions as a positive resource.

Robinson and Ward (1991) describe different models of resistance for African American female adolescents in a society that continually denigrates womanhood and blackness. They distinguish "resistance for survival" (personal, individualized, short-term survival strategies in the face of oppression) from "resistance for liberation and empowerment" (collective strategies whose goal is self-affirmation, self-determination, and community validation).[2] Robinson and Ward call on an Afrocentric model based on enhanced awareness of the strengths of African culture and tradition as a base for fostering positive resistance for liberation and empowerment. In thinking about Robinson and Ward's work, we have identified a third form of resistance, that of "resistance for

---

[2]During our monthly conversations, we also referred to this form of resistance as "resistance for transformation." This phrase occurs in Chapter 3.

equality." This form of resistance seeks equality under the law where diversity or difference does not lead to marginalization, inequality, and oppression, but rather equal opportunity and representation in all areas.

Finally, all of these ways of thinking about resistance have in common the view that women generate resistance out of their daily lives. Resistance, as Aptheker (1989) writes, "is about creating the conditions necessary for life, and it is about women expanding the limits of restrictions imposed upon them by misogynist, homophobic, racist, religious, and class boundaries" (p. 169).

Aptheker (1989) goes on to write that "women's resistance is not necessarily or intrinsically oppositional; it is not necessarily or intrinsically contesting for power. It does, however, have a profound impact on the fabric of social life because of its steady, cumulative effects. . . . To see women's resistance is also to see the accumulated effects of daily, arduous, creative, sometimes ingenious labors, performed over time, sometimes over generations" (p. 173).

All of the mothers in this book can teach us ways to observe resistance in daily life. Stacey (1997) describes a few strategies of resistance that are present in these chapters:

> Refusing to submit to other's pejorative definitions of oneself, is resis-
> tance. Being committed to living by modes of life and thought other
> than the dominant expectations...is resistance. Creating a counter-culture
> . . . is resistance. . . . Holding onto connections and relationships which
> problems endeavor to split apart, is resistance. Persisting with practicing
> one's non-dominant cultural knowledges and beliefs in the form of
> language, religion, health-care, community or family, is resistance. Forg-
> ing connections between other marginalized people whom the oppressor
> would have you believe are the "real" enemy, is resistance. Enduring
> on-going hardship while refusing to give up one's belief or life, is
> resistance. As a member of a marginalized culture, raising one's children
> to understand and to live in both their own and the dominant culture,
> is resistance. (p. 31)

It is our hope that the voices of the mothers in this book will contribute to our awareness of the ways in which mothers do resist the oppressive conditions of their lives, and that by noting these ways, we can contribute to processes whereby these daily acts of resistance become visible, gather mass, and count. We hope that these processes will transform the oppressive ideologies of motherhood into cultural practices that respect and support the multiplicity of ways that motherhood is lived.

## HOW THIS BOOK IS ORGANIZED

Bruner (1990) suggests that when there are breakdowns in a culture, or even a family, evidence for this can be noted in peoples' narratives. The "good mother" narrative shows signs of this. It is certainly an impoverished one. It attempts to assert uniformity where there is diversity; consensus where there are differing perspectives. We hope the individual chapters in this book will contribute a rich stock of maternal narratives that will create multiple centers and no edge.

Each chapter that follows speaks of a group of mothers whose lives or mothering practices are marginalized, and who have found ways to resist that marginalization. The individual stories are powerful, and so are the stories of each group.

Although the narrative of each diverse group of mothers is unique, we have come to see that there are also commonalities across groups. All of these mothers have experienced the pervasive processes of marginalization and tried in one way or another to put themselves at the center of their own narratives. For these reasons, groups that might initially be thought of as very dissimilar have much in common. In order to explore potential similarities across groups, we have arbitrarily arranged them into three clusters, Chapters 1–4, 5–8, and 9–12. Other, more intentional grouping schemas all seemed to reproduce the very marginalizing effect we were trying to critique. After the completed chapters were grouped in this way, the contributors to this book came together several times to take a broader view of each four-chapter cluster. Our aim was to identify unexpected points of convergence. These illuminating discussions were transcribed and edited into the "Conversations" that follow each cluster and comment upon the four chapters.

Since we started working on this book, many women have approached us with ideas for other chapters. We look forward to a book that includes the voices of many other groups of mothers, a book that will value their mothering practices and appreciate the contexts within which they mother. We hope that many others will take up the challenge of recognizing and respecting the daily acts of maternal resistance.

## REFERENCES

Aptheker, B. (1989). *Tapestries of life: Women's work, women's consciousness, and the meaning of daily experience.* Amherst, MA: University of Massachusetts Press.
Badinter, E. (1981). *Mother love: Myth and reality.* New York: Macmillan.

Bell-Scott, P., Guy-Sheftalle, B., Royster, J. J., Sims-Woods, J., DeCosta-Willis, M., & Fultz, L. P. (1991). *Double stitch: Black women write about mothers and daughters.* New York: HarperPerennial.

Block, R. H. (1978). American feminine ideals in transition: The rise of the moral mother, 1785–1815. *Feminist Studies, 4*(2), 101–126.

Braverman, L. (1989). Beyond the myth of motherhood. In M. McGoldrick, C. M. Anderson, & F. Walsh (Eds.), *Women and families: A framework for family therapy.* New York: Norton.

Bruner, J. (1990). *Acts of meaning.* Cambridge, MA: Harvard University Press.

Caplan, P., & Hall-McCorquodale, I. (1985). Mother-blaming in major clinical journals. *American Journal of Orthopsychiatry, 55,* 610–613.

Chodorow, N. J. (1978). *The reproduction of motherhood: Psychoanalysis and the sociology of gender.* Berkeley, CA: University of California Press.

Chodorow, N. J., & Contratto, S. (1982). The fantasy of the perfect mother. In B. Thorne with M. Yalom (Eds.), *Rethinking the family: Some feminist questions.* White Plains, NY: Longman Press.

Collins, P. H. (1987). The meaning of motherhood in Black culture and Black mother/daughter relationships. *Sage, 4*(2), 3–10.

Daly, B. O., & Reddy, M. T. (1991). *Narrating mothers: Theorizing maternal subjectivities.* Knoxville, TN: University of Tennessee Press.

Demos, J. (1983). The changing faces of fatherhood: A new exploration in family history. In F. Kessel & A. Siegel (Eds.), *The child and other cultural inventions.* New York: Praeger.

Ehrenreich, B., & English, D. (1979). *For her own good: 150 years of the experts' advice to women.* Garden City, NJ: Anchor Books.

Freire, P. (1989). *Pedagogy of the oppressed.* New York: Continuum.

García Coll, C., Cook-Nobles, R., & Surrey, J. L. (1995). *Diversity at the core: Implications for relational theory* (Working Paper Series No. 75). Wellesley, MA: Stone Center, Wellesley College.

Gilligan, C., Rogers, A. G., & Tolman, D. L. (Eds.). (1991). *Women, girls, and psychotherapy: Reframing resistance.* Binghamton, NY: Harrington Park Press.

Glenn, E. N., Chang, G., & Forcey, L. R. (1994). *Mothering: Ideology, experience, and agency.* New York: Routledge.

hooks, b. (1989). *Talking back: Thinking feminist, talking black.* Boston: South End Press.

Jordan, J., Kaplan, A., Miller, J. B., Stiver, I., & Surrey, J. L. (1991). *Women's growth in connection: Writings from the Stone Center.* New York: Guilford Press.

Knowles, J. P., & Cole, E. (1990). *Woman-defined motherhood.* Binghamton, NY: Harrington Park Press.

Margolis, M. L. (1984). *Mothers and such.* Berkeley, CA: University of California Press.

Miller, J. B. (1976). *Toward a new psychology of women.* Boston: Beacon Press.

Reddy, M. T., Roth, M., & Sheldon, A. (1994). *Mother journeys: Feminists write about mothering*. Minneapolis: Spinsters' Ink.

Robinson, T., & Ward, J. V. (1991). "A belief in self far greater than anyone's disbelief": Cultivating resistance among African American female adolescents. In C. Gilligan, A. G. Rogers, & D. L. Tolman (Eds.), *Women, girls, and psychotherapy: Reframing resistance*. Binghamton, NY: Harrington Park Press.

Stacey, K. (1997). Alternative metaphors for externalizing conversations. *Gecko, 1,* 29–51.

Surrey, J. L. (1990). Mother blaming and clinical theory. In J. P. Knowles & E. Cole (Eds.), *Motherhood: A feminist perspective*. New York: Haworth Press.

Surrey, J. L. (1996, May). *Relational and cultural constructions of motherhood: Clinical implications*. Lecture presented at Harvard Learning from Women Conference, Boston, MA.

Weingarten, K. (Ed.). (1995). *Cultural resistance: Challenging beliefs about men, women, and therapy*. New York: Haworth Press.

Weingarten, K. (1997). *The mother's voice: Strengthening intimacy in families*. New York: Guilford Press. (Originally published 1994 by Harcourt Brace)

Welch, S. (1985). *Communities of resistance and solidarity: A feminist theology of liberation*. New York: Orbis Books.

# 1

### Sidelined No More

#### Promoting Mothers of Adolescents as a
#### Resource for Their Growth and Development

*KATHY WEINGARTEN*

We live in a lattice of myths. Stories which
manifest the meaning of our lives and at the same
time define for us the circumference of the
imaginal world. What is it we are free to imagine?
—*SUSAN GRIFFIN, A Chorus of Stones*
(1992, p. 189)

*F O R* several years I have led workshops for clinicians on mothers and adolescent sons and daughters. Some of the participants are parenting an adolescent; most work with adolescents and their mothers in clinical or educational settings. Early in each workshop, I situate myself as the mother of an adolescent son[1] and daughter as well as a partisan zealot in my own self-imposed mission to change the cultural image of the mother–adolescent relationship. I ask people in the workshop to talk in pairs and tell a story of their own adolescence, preferably one that connects symbolically or literally to the time of their leaving home. I also request that the one who listens jot down words or phrases the speaker uses that seem particularly evocative to him or her. Following

[1]When I began these workshops my son was an adolescent. As of this writing, he is no longer a teen.

15

their talking in dyads, I collect the phrases that the notetakers have deemed significant.

Invariably, the same words repeat, whether the workshop is held in the deep South, the Midwest, the East or the West Coast. *Conflict* is the word that recurs most frequently. It is also the tone that pervades the words and phrases with which we paper the room. People offer words like these:

Challenging. Freedom. Difficult. Blocked. Confused. Disappointment. Devastation. Leaving. Anger. Abrupt transition. Intrusion. Ambivalence. Separate.

Recently, at one of these workshops, I asked people to identify themes in their stories. Through a process of sharing experiences of their adolescences, three ideas emerged. Conflict is inevitable. Distance is desirable. Separation is necessary. I then asked the workshop members to return to their dyads and talk about the effects of these ideas on their relationships with their mothers during adolescence. When we reconvened, people spoke with considerable poignancy about the effects that these ideas had had on their relational lives at adolescence. One man spoke particularly eloquently, expressing sadness and regret as he recollected that time 30 years ago:

> "I wanted to be close to my mother and that wish made me feel wrong and bad and stupid. At other times, I just felt confused about how I felt. I was never able to talk to my parents about what I was feeling—the fact that I felt lonely for them, but particularly my mother—because I thought I would be exposing something shameful."

This man's memory of his adolescent relationship with his mother fills him with sorrow now. Distance, not closeness, had characterized his relationship with his mother. Silence, not voice. Conflict, not carefree talk. The purpose of this chapter, like that of my workshop, is to identify the mechanisms that produce the perception and experience of adolescence as a time in which conflict, distance, and separation between teen and parent, particularly the mother, is inevitable. It is my further purpose to identify ways in which mothers and their adolescents, in conjunction with others, can resist the messages that create alienation and despair for mothers and teens just at the developmental moment when mutual knowing and collaboration become possible.

Throughout this chapter, much that I say about the cultural

messages that impinge on the mother–adolescent relationship will also be true about the father–adolescent relationship, for instance, messages about closeness, separation, and independence. Some messages, however, are uniquely directed to the mother–adolescent dyad, as some are to the father–adolescent dyad. Still others take on slightly different meanings when directed at mothers or fathers. My focus here is on mothers and mothering; I eagerly await scholarship that addresses the father–adolescent relationship from the perspective of the cultural messages that influence it.

How commonplace is it for cultural messages to infuse mother–adolescent interactions? Two anecdotes will illustrate this phenomenon. The first occurred a few years ago at a meeting of a Humanistic Jewish congregation during which teens who had made their bar and bat mitzvah recently were sharing portions of their speeches with the congregation members. Four young people spoke, apparently more briefly than the fifth young person had expected. Finding herself next in line, she aimed a confused and hapless expression at her mother. The mother walked up and whispered a suggestion to the daughter, who then turned to her text and began to read, seemingly helped by her mother's assistance. Some members of the audience, however, could not contain themselves enough to let the young woman carry on. Five or six comments were directed at the mother, in hushed voices, all of the ilk, "Don't you think she can take care of herself?" and "She wasn't worried; why were you?"

What stirred up some members of the audience to the degree that they violated the norms of the program by speaking out of turn? Having been a member of that audience, I saw nonverbal cues from the daughter to which the mother might have been responding. I know that I saw the daughter look at her mother, and I thought I saw an appeal in that look. I saw the mother respond quickly and relatively discreetly. It appeared to me that the daughter took the mother's suggestion. She regained her bearings and presented her bat mitzvah topic with clarity and sureness.

But what did other members of the audience see and react to? Some may not have believed that the daughter had looked to the mother for help. The comment "She wasn't worried . . . " suggests that not everyone did think the daughter was momentarily made anxious by the situation in which she unexpectedly found herself. To these audience members, the mother's response may have seemed intrusive, undermining, and smothering.

Underlying these differing perceptions, I believe, are differing calculations regarding the potential risks in this situation. I suspect that the mother thought that the main risk to her child lay in her experiencing confusion in front of an audience and, perhaps, in not "performing" as well as she might have. I suspect that some members of the audience felt that the main risk lay in the mother's "fixing" a situation that the daughter needed to handle by herself, thus undermining the daughter's sense of self-confidence.

The mother undoubtedly thought she was showing care; some members of the audience thought she should have let her daughter take care of herself. The mother probably thought that she was giving the daughter a small boost so that she could proceed independently. Those members of the audience who were aroused by the mother's behavior may have thought the mother was encouraging dependence. Some in the audience may have perceived the exchange as a demonstration of an admirable closeness and connection between the mother and daughter. Others may have thought they were looking at an example of a mother and adolescent pair who needed to work on separation.

All these themes and more are embedded in this seemingly simple event. What is central to this anecdote is that the mother's actions were denigrated and devalued, at least by those who commented. By deeming her actions inappropriate, they marginalized her mothering practice. It is the thesis of this chapter that mothers of adolescents are particularly vulnerable to having their mothering marginalized when they appear to violate white, Western, mainstream, mental health-sanctioned, middle-class norms regarding the importance of adolescence as a time to separate from the family, especially the mother.

Another anecdote will illustrate the point that mothering practices that seem to interfere with autonomy and independence and seem to compromise the developmental task of separation—for both mothers and adolescents—are harshly judged. The negative judgment is shaming to the mother and makes her action a source of worry, thus marginalizing it within her own repertoire of mothering practices.

I am a mother who has experienced the marginalization of her mothering practice. This next anecdote concerns myself and my son, Ben. In early winter of his freshman year in college, I received an e-mail from him saying that he had a cold and asking what he should do for it. I quickly responded and told him to do things I knew he knew to do, but that I knew would feel more comforting coming from me. "Drink plenty of fluids, rest, avoid milk products, and see if you can find chicken soup somewhere." By turn-around, I received another e-mail: "Thanks. I'm not eating chicken anymore. Now what?"

A few hours later, I happened to be speaking to a friend who informed me that Ben was having dinner with her the following night. Not thinking anything of it, I said to her, the mother of two adult daughters, "He's not eating chicken anymore," to which she crisply responded, "He can tell me that himself."

What was my friend reacting to? Was her response simply critical or also protective, and of whom? A seasoned mother who is 10 years ahead of me in navigating the developmental transition from adolescence to young adult, was she trying to protect Ben from my meddling or to steer me to a less-involved maternal position?

Her response implied that my behavior had violated a boundary. Ben should be the *only* one to tell people about matters of concern to him, perhaps especially dietary ones. In the short sequence between my friend and me, I felt that the richness of my relationship with Ben was capsized into a narrow cultural precept: Mothers must back off and let their children be independent at adolescence. I wanted Ben to be independent and hadn't thought my comment would compromise his efforts. My friend, obviously, saw the comment as part of a pattern that could.

Her message was consistent with that delivered by many people, representing many different institutions—for example, the family, schools, and the health care industry. The message—back off—obscures our ability to consider together what we mean by independence and how we think young people achieve it. The message seems to value separation above all else at this time in the family life cycle. My point is that there are other options at this time; separation is not the be-all and end-all of the mother–adolescent task.

## THE DISCOURSE OF MOTHERS AND ADOLESCENCE

How did the message about separation come to be so ubiquitous? To understand this nearly universal prescription for adolescents and their mothers, I rely on the framework of discourse analysis. I am using the concept of discourse the way social historian Joan W. Scott defines it, that is, discourse is a "historically, socially, and institutionally specific structure of statements, terms, categories, and beliefs" (Scott, 1990, pp. 135–136) that are embedded in institutions, social relationships, and texts. Some discourses are dominant and others are marginalized through the operation of these mechanisms. This meaning of discourse allows us to make sense of what Jerome Bruner calls the ways "culture forms mind" (Bruner, 1990, p. 24). At the same time, it is important to remember that we live in multiple cultural contexts simultaneously and that the discourses that influence us reflect the multiplicity of cultures within which we live.

In other work, I have written at length about the discourse of mothers (Weingarten, 1995b, 1997b). The one characteristic that I found in my research was that in every culture and in every era there was a dominant prescription of what constituted "good" and "bad" mothering. Though what was coded as good or bad varied, the fact of coding was universal (see Introduction, this volume).

### "Bad" Moms

In a recent cartoon by Roz Chast (1996), the idea of the bad mother merges with the symbolism of the baseball card to show that blaming mother is as American as apple pie. Chast proposes that people can collect "Bad Mom Cards," and then depicts nine moms whose behavior has crossed the ideological divide between good and bad. The text for Card #39: Dawn K, for example, reads, "When daughter left stuffed bear in Grand Union, waited until *next day* to retrieve it." Each card simultaneously attests to while it mocks the very standards it exposes. Chast makes it plain that no behavior is too trivial to escape assignment into the ubiquitous good–bad categories.

In this cartoon all the moms are white. While discussing the significance of this fact in a class of mine, one African American mom suggested that white Americans' knowledge of African American mothers is so limited that in their imagination no bad behavior of the African American mother is trivial, thus the premise of the cartoon would fail. For instance, "Paulette K: 'Let her kids play on the sidewalk after dark' " isn't funny. The stakes are too high. But, by knowing more about African American lives, white Americans could be amused by "Gave her kids grits 5 days in a row."

Chast's cartoon suggests that no mothering practice is immune from scrutiny. Mothers, however, vary considerably in the extent to which they are vulnerable to the perpetual gaze and vulnerable to seeing themselves as bad mothers. Some mothers seem mired in their perception of their "evilness," whereas others seem oblivious to any faults. Still others judge their every thought and deed, whereas others are satisfied to do the best they can. Despite a range of responses, all mothers are made vulnerable by the good–bad split.

## "Good" Moms

Despite dramatic shifts that place more North American mothers of young children in the workforce than at home, the definition of a "good" mother retains its turn-of-the-century stamp: The good mother holds herself primarily responsible for raising healthy, well-adjusted children (Thurer, 1994). As Joan W. Scott (1990) describes, this message is embedded in texts, relationships, and institutions. For instance, there are thousands of popular magazines and books directed toward mothers, and, less frequently, mothers and fathers, on how to teach, improve, or help their children. The embedded message is that the good mother holds herself responsible for raising productive children and will do whatever she needs to do to accomplish this goal.

The message is embedded in relationships in overt and covert ways. In the following example, a message about mothers is embedded covertly. It is common for teachers who know nothing of a child's family structure to say to children, "Take this paper home and have your mother sign it." The teacher is assuming that each child has a home with one mother and that she is the person who handles the school–family interface.

Finally, messages about what constitutes a good mother are embedded in institutional mandates and regulations, such as those used by departments of social services in their definitions of abuse and neglect and by courts in deciding custody of children. For example, in 1991 the California Court of Appeals ruled on the request of a woman who had carried the fertilized egg and sperm of a married couple to a term birth to be declared the baby's "natural" mother and to be allowed visitation rights. The judge declared that as the "gestational" carrier of the child, the woman was merely a "host" and had no legal standing to the child (Annas, 1992). In effect, the judge ruled on a definition of the good mother: She is a married woman and not a young, single woman like the "host."

## "Good" Moms of Adolescents

In this discourse, the dominant message about goodness of mothers assumes a young child, not an adolescent (Berry, 1993). As the child grows, the dominant message prescribing the feelings, attitudes, and behavior of the good mother shifts substantially. With regard to an adolescent, a mother's involvement is easily defined as intrusion, care as invasion of privacy, and responsibility as overprotection. Only those behaviors, attitudes, and feelings that support separation are considered legitimate (Lazarre, 1991).

Often the embedded message is revealed through absence. It is as meaningful to interpret the absence of images or writing about mothers and adolescents as it is necessary to interpret what is present, for example, in art forms and print (Weingarten, 1995a). There are relatively few images that show adolescents with their mothers. Ads rarely show a teen with a mother or show older women with younger women or men, for that matter. Contemporary movies, for instance, the 1995 hits *Clueless* and *Kids,* don't even depict teens as having mothers. Books for parents of teens sport 100 ways to back off gracefully. High schools rarely have programming that involves mothers, or fathers, with their teens (Carnegie Council on Adolescent Development, 1995). Even at school sporting events, it is rare to see an adolescent sitting with her or his mother. The absence of images of mothers with adolescent sons or daughters signifies the relative lack of importance mainstream culture attaches to the mother's role at this time in the life cycle.

Perhaps most striking is the difficulty of stating what is valued about the mother of an adolescent. How is the "good" mother of the adolescent son or daughter described? What does she do that is desirable? Keep the refrigerator stocked? Accommodate large groups of friends in the house? Is the mother present when the food is consumed and the friends are entertained, or does she stay in the background, out of the way? The paucity of imagery and popular lore about what the "good" mother of an adolescent does points, I believe, to the central tasks to which the mother of the adolescent is supposed to devote herself. The "good" mother of an adolescent son or daughter supports distance between them, accepts conflict, and encourages their separation from her.

## Distance

The culture at large is promoting one developmental goal for adolescents: separation (Dickerson & Zimmerman, 1992, 1993). To promote this goal, distance is necessary. However, the very distance that adolescents and their mothers "negotiate" may actually create more problems at this stage than gains. Few adolescents are mature enough actually to live apart from their parents, and most adolescents intuit this. The conflict that often occurs between parent and teen, mother and son or daughter, may be a manifestation of the bind that the young persons find themselves in. If the successful teen is one who is independent of her or his parents and the successful mother is the one who gives her teen "space," then how do they manage the very real needs that the young person has? They do so often in conflict.

## Conflict

The dominant cultural image of adolescent and mother is adversarial, and the deck is stacked for the teen to win. The culture wants teens to win, and the prize is their independence. For the teen to win, in this paradigm, the mother must lose both status and authority. Mothers must be sidelined if they don't sideline themselves. Mothers are viewed as the very persons from whom teens must separate to achieve a culturally sanctioned imprimatur of success (Apter, 1990).

## Separation

Achieving separation, the wider culture would have it, is the gold standard of success for adolescents. Mothers are depicted as most likely to stand in the adolescent's way. Robert Bly, a chief spokesman for the contemporary men's movement, is perhaps as vehement and graphic as any writer about this goal for boys. In *Iron John: A Book about Men,* his best-selling work describing a boy's journey to manhood, he writes:

> The traditional initiation break is clearly preferable, and sidesteps the violence. But all over the country now one sees hulking sons acting ugly in the kitchen and talking rudely to their mothers, and I think it's an attempt to make themselves unattractive. If the old men haven't done their work to interrupt the mother–son unity, what else can the boys do to extricate themselves but to talk ugly? . . . A clean break from the mother is crucial. (Bly, 1990, p. 19)

Why is a clean break thought crucial, not just for sons but for daughters as well? I think at the heart of the matter is a confusion between separation and differentiation and, perhaps even more importantly, confusion about what intimacy is. Too often people think that intimacy is synonymous with closeness and then worry that mother–son or mother–daughter closeness will obstruct the young person's development.

What does the language of closeness conjure up that is disturbing? For boys, one objection, I think, is a political one. Boys mustn't remain close to their mothers because mothers are not the people from whom boys can learn how to take their proper place in the social order. Because boys must be able to dominate women, and because mothers are "superior" to sons in the generational hierarchy, closeness to the mother will produce unworkable binds for the mother–son relationship. Distance is the preferred solution. Daughters, on the other hand, can stay close because their "proper" place is precisely to learn from their mothers how to tend to hearth and home.

A second basis for objection is sexual. Mothers and sons must put distance between them at puberty to control the sexual attractions between them. Shades of Oedipus and Jocasta. Yet intertwined with concern for potential sexual impropriety may lurk another layer of distress. In a sexual encounter with his mother, an adolescent boy would not be the dominant partner—as a male "should" be in a sexual encounter; his mother would be. This adds a political dimension to the feared sexual violation.

Curiously, mother–daughter closeness doesn't seem to conjure up the same kind of sexual worry in most people. I suspect that the absence of a clear prohibition or even concern reflects a deep-seated homophobia based on a denial of sexual desire between women. Clearly, I am not advocating sexual intimacy between mothers and their sons or daughters, but only observing how different the concern over closeness between mothers and sons seems to be from that over mothers and daughters.

Mother–daughter closeness seems to be of concern because there is an assumption that the mother is gratifying her needs at the expense of the daughter's. The presumption is that closeness between mother and daughter invariably masks a mother's dependence on her daughter, a dependence that inevitably compromises the daughter's independence.

Reconceptualizing intimacy as something more complex than closeness is a strategy aimed at the production of cultural messages. It is my hope that if we can come to think about intimacy differently, sons and daughters will be "released" to be in relationships with their mothers. Relationship, not a "clean break," is crucial for teens if they are to become able citizens of our complex world, for it is their mothers who are in the best position to assist teens in developing the independence skills they need to function competently. It is relationship, not separation, that will bring mothers of adolescents back from the periphery of their children's lives into the center, a center in which they coexist harmoniously with peers and other adults (Jordan, Kaplan, Miller, Stiver, & Surrey, 1991). Only when mothers are seen as also vital to the development of their adolescent children's lives will the marginalization of mothers of teens stop (Blakeley, 1994; Silverstein & Rashbaum, 1994).

## INTIMACY

The reconceptualization of intimacy that I am proposing begins with thinking about intimacy in terms of moments of connection, moments, for instance, when I feel that I have shared something that is important to me and the other person has listened and understood me (Weingarten, 1991, 1997b). Or, reciprocally, intimacy develops when someone shares something with me and I have listened well and respectfully to that person. For me, intimacy is about sharing feelings, thoughts, wishes, and activities.

I think of intimacy as something that people can create with each other at any time, if they are open to sharing what they truly care about with each other and to trying to understand what the other finds meaningful. Intimacy protects people against pain and fosters self-knowledge. Intimacy promotes differentiation, that refinement of self-awareness that creates emotional sturdiness. Finally intimacy supports action when needed. With this view of intimacy, distance is not desirable, conflict is not inevitable, and separation may interfere with differentiation.

Rather than thinking of intimacy as desirable but difficult to accomplish, I have a rock-bottom faith that it is achievable . . . with the right kind of effort. Part of that effort is resisting the idea that boys have less capacity for intimacy than girls, and resisting the idea that girls who are intimate with their mothers are emotionally fused with them.

### The Gender Story

Where is it written that boys are less capable of intimacy than girls? It is written in many places. I call this a "gender story." According to this story, boys are considered less able to develop intimate relationships than girls, mothers are discouraged from sustaining intimate relationships with sons past puberty, and mother–daughter intimacy is touted as having "the materials for the deepest mutuality and the most painful estrangement" (Rich, 1986, p. 226).

Nancy Chodorow, a psychoanalytically oriented sociologist, may be the most frequently cited exponent of a theory that posits a gendered capacity for intimacy. In her widely acclaimed book, *The Reproduction of Mothering,* Chodorow (1978) attempts to account for the way modern capitalist society creates and re-creates feminine and masculine personalities such that women will be suited to mother and men will be suited to work in the alienating structures of capitalism. Using object relations and Marxism as her primary theories, she identifies the near universality of female responsibility for childcare—rather than biological, cultural, or economic factors—as the reason for consistent gendered personality differences.

Focusing on the first 3 years of life, Chodorow (1978) states that growing girls come to define themselves as like their mothers whom they observe relating intimately with them. Boys, on the other hand, come to define themselves as separate and distinct from their mothers, thus making intimate relationships appear to be something females but not males care about or nurture. Chodorow believes that this early difference predisposes girls to have greater potential than boys for participating in intimate relationships.

Further, Chodorow (1978) believes that mothers experience their sons as more different from themselves than daughters, more "other." She believes that mothers' differential responses to their male and female children integrally contribute to what turns out to be a cycle in which mothering exclusively by females reproduces the capacity to mother—to be intimate—in daughters but not sons.

This observation has functioned as much like a prescription as a description. Absorbed by popular culture, reflecting preexisting cultural premises as well as shaping new ones, the idea that mothers and sons do not, should not, cannot be as intimate as mothers and daughters has had destructive consequences.

These destructive consequences play themselves out in small and great ways. Whether we want to or not, many mothers, myself included, receive the message to pull away from our sons and enact it daily, in both trivial and significant ways. We pause. I fear that the accumulation of just such moments of pausing may have dire consequences for mothers and sons. Personally and professionally, we are bombarded with messages that pathologize mother–son closeness. We are directed to see involvement as inevitably undermining autonomy. What we don't see is that mothers are being directed to abandon their sons too soon. Mothers and sons, however, need to feel entitled to sustained, nonintrusive, nonsexualized intimacy in order to work for it.

The same is true for mothers and daughters. Although I do not think that mothers of daughters are encouraged to pull away from them to the extent that mothers are encouraged to do so with sons, there is still the same failure to identify benefits from mother–daughter intimacy.

Since the early 1980s, the work of the Stone Center group (Bergman, 1991; Jordan et al., 1991) has challenged and expanded these formulations deriving from object relations theory. Favoring an exploration of connection rather than a (too narrow) focus on separation, they have developed theory to account for "growth in connection," growth in relationships for both girls and boys, men and women. My work on intimacy, a form of connection, has points in common with the pathbreaking work of Judith Jordan, Alexandra Kaplan, Jean Baker Miller, Irene Stiver, and Janet Surrey.

In my redefinition of intimacy, in which intimacy is viewed as moments of interaction in which there is mutual meaning making, sustaining intimacy does not require continuous intimate experience. This model of intimacy, I believe, fits the usual relationship between mothers and their adolescent sons and daughters well, relationships in which intermittency is customary. Episodic intimate interaction serves growth and development; it does not undermine it.

## CLINICAL ILLUSTRATION

To accomplish intimacy between mother and teen requires that they both consider the mother a person who has a life story as compelling as her child's, one with as much potential for transformation. When the culture—both local and at large—assists rather than undermines intimacy between mother and teens, both benefit from sharing the truths of their lives.

A recent consultation that I did with two mothers and their daughters dramatically demonstrated the power of both teen and mother speaking in each other's presence (Weingarten, 1997a). The effect of the speaking had both short- and long-term impact, both of which I will recount briefly.

I was asked to consult with two mothers and their teenaged daughters by the director of an inpatient residence for problem adolescents (Nichols & Jacques, 1995). Both girls had a history of running away from the residence and placing themselves in high-risk situations. The two mother–daughter pairs were apprehensive about the format; neither the girls nor their mothers knew each other well, nor had the mothers and daughters been successful in the past at staying in the room together during conjoint therapy appointments.

I saw my task as that of creating opportunities for the mothers and daughters to talk about their lives in ways that discouraged defensiveness. I needed my questions to create a parallel universe of assumptions to the ones in which these mothers and daughters—as are all mothers and daughters—were drenched.

Overall, I hoped that the interview would make material the following ideas:

- Daughters can listen to mothers.
- Mothers have stories too.
- Sharing intimately does not undermine generational boundaries.
- Intimacy is built up of shared meanings.
- A goal of conversation can be mutual understanding, not agreement.
- Mother blaming is counterproductive; mothers are not responsible for all the problems in their children's lives (Caplan, 1989).
- Adolescents do want to be understood by adults and maintain connections with them.
- Adults can change. Adults can develop personal resources they didn't have before.
- Community is an available resource for everybody.

The two mothers, Bonnie, age 34, and Roberta, age 32, though anxious, were cooperative and eager to begin talking about the girls' problems. Bonnie's daughter, Maryann, a slightly built 16-year-old, huddled in her chair, looking as if she were trying to take up as little space as possible. Tara, age 12, Roberta's daughter, had a robust, healthy appearance, but she too sat with her back pushed into the chair, and let her long blond hair cover her face much of the time.

At first I asked general questions to get to know the bare facts of their lives and to set out my expectations for the interview. Several minutes into the conversation, Maryann volunteered that she had known she was in trouble long before anyone else had noticed, at age 11. Her evidence was her drinking, depression, and suicidality. With great sadness, she indicated that no one noticed her trouble until she stopped going to school at age 14½.

Maryann's description was clearly painful for her mother to hear but she sat listening to Maryann intently, without challenging her or defending herself. I wondered aloud about how old Tara had been when she knew she was in trouble.

"Me? Trouble? I was 4. I was hanging around people who were smoking joints and doing drugs."

Roberta hadn't noticed that Tara was in trouble because she too had been in trouble. At this point in the interview, I was weaving among the four women's stories of their lives, of the trouble they were in, and the reasons behind it. Roberta had been in trouble with drugs and drinking since age 9. Later in the interview she revealed that her stepfather had abused her between the ages of 9 and 17, which was the reason for her trouble, she maintained.

Bonnie, too, had been in trouble with drinking and drugs. She had been 15 when her trouble began, and no one had noticed. Moments later in the interview, she told us that her mother had died the year before she got into trouble and that her father had been drunk all the time.

"Would things have been different for you if your mother had lived?"

"Absolutely."

Maryann was clear, however, that they wouldn't have been different for her because her mother "married an asshole." She went on to explain. Maryann had also been abused by her stepfather, and, later, Tara revealed that there had been "trouble" between her and one of her mother's boyfriends.

Realizing that our time was nearly over, I moved to summarize what I had heard and to propose that we think together about what ideas people had "to break the pattern."

Tara spoke first. "We just talk about it. Like at birthday parties, my aunts and us, and the guys too, we talk about it. Sometimes we try to get my grandmother to talk about it, but she never wants to."

"So talking about it. Facing it helps," I said.

Roberta then spoke definitely. "Recovery."

Maryann was looking far off, and I wondered aloud if this was making any sense to her. She said it was, but it didn't matter. Nothing mattered anymore.

The other women chimed in. They knew how Maryann felt. Her heart, they said, is cold, it can't feel.

Drawing a large heart on the easel, I turned to Maryann and asked if she would draw a line to show us how much of her heart was warm, how much cold. Slowly, she left her seat, and drew a line showing that more of her heart was cold and without feeling. Still, it was significant that a part of her still did have feeling.

The moment felt sacred. Bonnie spoke first. "I think it has to do with care. I think that if they feel that nobody cares, then that's where the not feeling comes in."

"But both of you moms do care," I said with some urgency in my voice.

"But they don't feel it," Bonnie explained to me. "Because our caring is cold caring, because of the way we were brought up."

"Right," Roberta joined in emphatically.

"So we can sit here and say we care, but it may not be enough of a feeling because we don't even know what it feels like," continued Bonnie.

Now Roberta, Bonnie, and I started talking. I asked them what might happen if they had a mother's group in which they could learn from each other how to show warm care? They agreed it might help.

There were only a few minutes left. Roberta was tearful. "I'm willing to do anything to help Tara, to help me, to help the generations. I don't want her life to be anything like mine, with the pain, the using, the not liking myself, and the insecurity. It feels good that you guys shared with us."

Tara and Maryann demurred, but Bonnie had a lot to say. "It's great to know we're not alone. Other people are going through similar things. To learn the causes of why things happened and to realize that I'm not to blame. I can see why I did things. All this time I've really been blaming myself for screwing up, and now I know why I did. Now maybe it will make it easier for me to connect with Maryann knowing that our paths really aren't that different."

During this interview the four women did experience linkages in their paths, and this had immediate repercussions. Several months after this interview, Bonnie and Roberta asked the residence director to call me and tell me what had happened since we had met.

The mothers said they felt less blamed and had more energy to work with their daughters. They were finding the support of other mothers in the parents' group that they started invaluable. Finally they said that the interview had helped them "know stuff we knew but didn't know we knew."

I wrote them immediately thanking them for sharing these events with me and letting them know that their sharing had affected me both personally and professionally. I wanted them to know that their responses had further convinced me of the value of mothers sharing themselves with their daughters and daughters doing so with their mothers.

In the interview with Bonnie and Roberta, Maryann and Tara, I acted to discredit a primary cultural assumption that mothers cannot be a resource for their adolescent children. On the contrary, believing that adolescents can benefit from knowing their mothers, even when their mothers have troubled pasts, I facilitated a conversation in which all four women realized that they had some common problems and some common ideas about solutions to them. Mutual knowing, not separation; independence skills, not autonomy were the precepts that guided my interaction with the four.

In a follow-up interview with Bonnie and Roberta 2 years later, both mothers felt more optimistic about their relationships with their daughters; both were in genuine dialogues. The two mothers felt empowered by their new positions with their daughters and able to do more for themselves and their daughters with their new sense of confidence. Roberta's and Bonnie's experiences are replicable. When mothers are honored as resources for their teens, they become more fully participatory in their own lives as well. This outcome is good for mothers, good for their children, and good for the community.[2]

## TAKING THE POSITION PUBLICLY: WHAT PROFESSIONALS AND MOTHERS CAN DO

### Clinical Work

Clinical wisdom about adolescence views psychological separation as one of the essential tasks of this time period, both reflecting and reinforcing the cultural beliefs about its desirability. The therapeutic challenge for the therapist is thus conceptualized as a paradox: "The adolescent must seek help from a person whom he links with those internal parental representations from which he is trying to emancipate himself" (Jaffe & Offer, 1980, p. 308). Therapists are advised to "dissociate" themselves from parents' behavior to manage this dilemma.

Although family meetings are encouraged in working with adolescents, parents are not seen as resources but rather as people who have

---

[2]For a more detailed case report, including an edited transcript of the session, see Weingarten (1997a).

contributed to the adolescents' difficulties. In a section of a review article on the role of the family in the treatment of adolescents, not a single positive dimension of the parents' role is listed (Jaffe & Offer, 1980).

Current views of the parents' role in the treatment of their adolescent may be shifting. In a more recent review article, clinicians were advised to find ways of integrating parents into the child's therapy (Kovacs & Lohr, 1995). These authors acknowledge that the omission of parents from the treatment process "diminishes their educational and psychological importance" (Kovacs & Lohr, 1995, p. 20).

However, there is still concern about protecting the confidentiality of the adolescent. This also produces dilemmas. All too frequently therapists manage this dilemma by creating a rigid boundary between themselves and the parent, usually the mother. When mothers try to find out what is happening with their child, therapists often blame mothers for being intrusive. This intrusiveness confirms the therapist's original operating assumption, but the therapist may fail to see how it was a self-fulfilling prophecy.

An alternative clinical view would take as its starting point that mothers can be the most powerful therapeutic resource adolescents have. In fact, a three-decade longitudinal study of all children born on the island of Kauai, Hawaii, in 1955 found three factors strongly associated with resilience in high-risk individuals, the second of which was strong attachments with parents or parental substitutes (Werner & Smith, 1992). Clinicians could work toward defusing conflict, promoting understanding, and developing strategies for mothers to assist their adolescents with the very real struggles they have, be they related to issues with peers, school, self-esteem, sexuality, or violence. Clinical work based on the Stone Center model of growth in connection would offer numbers of ideas for working with mothers and their adolescent sons and daughters from the perspective of strengthening the relationship between them (Jordan et al., 1991).

Clinicians can also encourage the creation of "teams" for mothers and adolescents. Many of the difficulties adolescents face, which therefore their mothers also face at this stage, are problems for which support from others may be critical at times. Clinicians can help mothers and teens identify who in their networks might act as members of a support team, like a pit crew, to add a little extra perspective, comfort, or help when times are tough (Steinberg, 1990; Weingarten & Worthen, 1997; White, 1995). The goal is not only to help adolescents but to improve the overall health of families and communities.

## Schools

Clinicians are not the only ones who are in a position to foster ties between mothers and teens. School personnel are uniquely placed to promote cooperation and collaboration between mothers and adolescents. Instead, all too often, school programming divides parents and teens, leaving the sidelines as the only place for parents to cheer on, but not participate in, their children's activities.

The Carnegie Council on Adolescent Development documents that parental involvement declines steadily as children move through middle and upper schools (1995, p. 12). Schools do not provide parents with clear outlets for their interest in staying involved with their children as they advance through school, or, at best, they provide parents with opportunities to work on behalf of the student community rather than with their own children.

Change is urgently needed. Mothers, and fathers too, have much to contribute to schools as well as to learn. To teach teens effectively, the people they live with must be "on board." Outreach to parents may be indicated, and, in some instances, parallel instruction could be offered to ensure that parents will be supporters rather than detractors of the school curricula.

Programming shifts would be easy to accomplish; it is the belief system that provides the rationale for the programming that must change. This change would need to start in the schools that train teachers and middle and high school administrators.

## Health Care

Change is also needed in the delivery of health care services to adolescents. In most health care systems, early adolescence heralds the moment when children are seen by themselves, and their parents are excluded from the exam and often the discussion of the relevant medical issues, be they related to a medical problem or a health behavior such as weight and eating, sexual behavior, smoking and substance use, and so forth. Clearly adolescents—like all people—need privacy, but early adolescence is a critical time for disease prevention and health promotion education. Parents, especially mothers, should be critical components in any integrated disease prevention/health promotion plan. Medical personnel may need simultaneously to instruct mothers in disease prevention and health promotion strategies. This will not only affect compliance rates for teens but also improve the health of their mothers.

## CONCLUSION

I am proposing that mothers be treated as allies, not obstacles, in the lives of their adolescent sons and daughters. To do so requires reconceptualizing adolescent and maternal development. Mothers can no longer be seen as selfless vessels whose job it is to be receptive to whatever their adolescents want to dump on them or fill them with. Adolescents can no longer be seen as quixotic characters, victims of their own hormones and responsive only to a peer culture manipulated by greedy media. We must assume instead that adolescents want to retain positive connections with their mothers and will appreciate it if the major institutions in their lives encourage rather than undermine these relationships. We must assume too that mothers of adolescents have compelling lives of their own and that their wishes to be involved in their adolescents' lives stem from appropriate concern, not inappropriate boundaries.

In the workshops on adolescents and their mothers that I mentioned in the beginning of this paper, I ask participants who have spent the day learning new conceptualizations of mother–son and mother–daughter connection to reimagine their own relationships with their mothers. I ask them what words or phrase would describe their preferred relationship. By the end of the day the words and phrases have shifted significantly: open sharing. Coming and going is lifelong. Elasticity between generations. Growing up is lifelong. Separation isn't frightening. Connection with others is possible. Mutual appreciation. Mutual enhancement. Evolving toward more richness. Looping back and forth between parent and teen. Support for a healthy transition.

The man who had spoken about his distant relationship with his mother had much to say. He said he understood now that his confusion was produced by his having had ideas that conflicted with the dominant discourse of mothers and adolescent sons. Confusion had stopped him from sharing ideas that might have been considered odd or even pathological. Invited to imagine the relationship he would have wanted to have with his mother, he described one in which mutual closeness, honesty, respect, and interest prevailed. "I can work for this in other lives," he said. "With the families I treat and with my own children. I believe that intimacy is possible and desirable between mothers and their sons and daughters."

As mothers and as professionals we should wish and work for no less.

## REFERENCES

Annas, G. J. (1992). Using genes to define motherhood: The California solution. *New England Journal of Medicine, 326,* 417–420.

Apter, T. (1990). *Altered loves: Mothers and daughters during adolescence.* New York: St. Martin's Press.

Bergman, S. (1991). *Men's psychological development: A relational perspective.* Wellesley, MA: Stone Center, Wellesley College.

Berry, M. F. (1993). *The politics of parenthood: Child care, women's rights, and the myth of the good mother.* New York: Penguin Books.

Blakeley, M. K. (1994). *American mom: Motherhood, politics, and humble pie.* New York: Workman.

Bly, R. (1990). *Iron John: A book about men.* Reading, MA: Addison-Wesley.

Bruner, J. (1990). *Acts of meaning.* Cambridge, MA: Harvard University Press.

Caplan, P. (1989). *Don't blame mother. Mending the mother–daughter relationship.* New York: HarperCollins.

Carnegie Council on Adolescent Development. (1995). *Great transitions: Preparing adolescents for a new century.* New York: Carnegie.

Chast, R. (1996, February 26 and March 4). Bad mom cards. *The New Yorker,* p. 153.

Chodorow, N. (1978). *The reproduction of mothering: Psychoanalysis and the sociology of gender.* Berkeley, CA: University of California Press.

Dickerson, V. C., & Zimmerman, J. L. (1992). Families with adolescents: Escaping problem lifestyles. *Family Process, 31,* 341–353.

Dickerson, V. C., & Zimmerman, J. L. (1993). A narrative approach to families with adolescents. In S. Friedman (Ed.), *The new language of change: Constructive collaboration in psychotherapy.* New York: Guilford Press.

Griffin, S. (1992). *A chorus of stones: The private life of war.* New York: Doubleday.

Jaffe, C., & Offer, D. (1980). Psychotherapy with adolescents. In G. P. Sholevar (Ed.), *Emotional disorders in children and adolescents: Medical and psychological approaches to treatment.* New York: Spectrum.

Jordan, J. V., Kaplan, A. G., Miller, J. B., Stiver, I. P., & Surrey, J. L. (1991). *Women's growth in connection: Writings from the Stone Center.* New York: Guilford Press.

Kovacs, M., & Lohr, W. D. (1995). Research on psychotherapy with children and adolescents: An overview of evolving trends and current issues. *Journal of Abnormal Child Psychology, 23*(1), 11–30.

Lazarre, J. (1991). *Worlds beyond my control.* New York: Dutton.

Nichols, T., & Jacques, C. (1995). Family reunions: Communities celebrate new possibilities. In S. Friedman (Ed.), *The reflecting team in action: Collaborative practice in family therapy.* New York: Guilford Press.

Rich, A. (1986). *Of woman born* (10th anniversary ed.). New York: Norton.

Scott, J. W. (1990). Deconstructing equality-versus-difference: Or, the uses of poststructuralist theory for feminism. In M. Hirsch & E. F. Keller (Eds.), *Conflicts in feminism.* New York: Routledge.

Silverstein, O., & Rashbaum, B. (1994). *The courage to raise good men.* New York: Viking.

Steinberg, L. (1990). Autonomy, conflict, and harmony in the family relationship. In S. S. Feldman & G. R. Elliott (Eds.), *At the threshold: The developing adolescent.* Cambridge, MA: Harvard University Press.

Thurer, S. (1994). *The myths of motherhood: How culture reinvents the good mother.* Houghton Mifflin.

Weingarten, K. (1991). The discourses of intimacy: Adding a social constructionist and feminist view. *Family Process, 31,* 285–305.

Weingarten, K. (1995a). Introduction: Attending to absence. In K. Weingarten (Ed.), *Cultural resistance: Challenging beliefs about men, women, and therapy.* New York: Haworth Press.

Weingarten, K. (1995b). Radical listening: Challenging cultural beliefs for and about mothers. In K. Weingarten (Ed.), *Cultural resistance: Challenging beliefs about men, women, and therapy.* New York: Haworth Press.

Weingarten, K. (1997a). From "cold care" to "warm care": Challenging the discourses of mothers and adolescents. In C. Smith & D. Nylund (Eds.), *Narrative therapies with children and adolescents.* New York: Guilford Press.

Weingarten, K. (1997b). *The mother's voice: Strengthening intimacy in families.* New York: Guilford Press. (Originally published 1994 by Harcourt Brace)

Weingarten, K., & Worthen, M. E. W. (1997). A narrative approach to understanding the illness experiences of a mother and daughter. *Families, Systems and Health, 15,* 41–54.

Werner, E. E., & Smith, R. S. (1992). *Overcoming the odds: High-risk children from birth to adulthood.* Ithaca, NY: Cornell University Press.

White, M. (1995). *Re-authoring lives: Interviews and essays.* Adelaide, Australia: Dulwich Centre Publications.

# 2

## "Exceptional" Mothering in a "Normal" World

*MIRIAM GREENSPAN*

A S the mother of a child with disabilities, I read with particular interest Beverly Lowry's review of a book by Michael Berube called *Life as We Know It: A Father, a Family, and an Exceptional Child* in *The New York Times Book Review*. The review starts off: "Some things having to do with children the heart can barely stand. When we read or hear stories telling of such things—parental neglect, parental brutality, babies born addicted to cocaine, political torture . . . we can only lower our eyes and wish for life to be otherwise" (Lowry, *The New York Times Book Review*, October 27, 1996, p. 22). Before reading this book, the reviewer admits, she would have "slotted Down Syndrome into that list of unthinkables."

My daughter Esther does not have Down syndrome, but she is a child who is visibly "different." In the 10 years of her life, I have never thought to associate her with political torture or parental brutality. When I look into her loving, sparkling blue eyes, I don't see something "unthinkable." I had Esther, my third child, when I was 39 years old. I intentionally chose not to do a "routine" amniocentesis, though I knew first hand that not all babies are born "normal." My first child, Aaron, had severe medical problems at birth and died at 2 months. Anna, my second child, was born radiantly healthy. I have the old-fashioned idea that the child that comes to me is the child I am entrusted to love, and I have chosen to leave my fate as a mother in the lap of nature, rather than in the machinery of medical technology. I have no regrets, despite knowing what I know about the sorrows of raising a child with disabilities.

On the other hand, what *my* heart can barely stand is the fact that many people, like this reviewer, find "different" children "unthinkable" and indeed "lower their eyes" at the sight or thought of them—an apt image for the shunning of disabled people and their families. Her words reflect our society's fundamental fear of "difference." Disabilities like Down syndrome are lumped together with political torture and parental brutality presumably because they are all painful and beyond the pale of "normal life." But the fact is that disabilities (and all sorts of other "unthinkables") are very much a part of normal life—a part designated as "abnormal" and thereby ghettoized socially, fiscally, institutionally, and emotionally from the "mainstream." If they are unthinkable it's because we are unwilling or unable to think about them. One result is the isolation and marginalization of families with special needs.

Webster's definition of "margin" includes "the outside limit and adjoining surface of something: edge" as well as "measure or degree of difference." "Marginalization," a word not to be found in my dictionary, has to do with being shunted to the outer edge of the social mainstream because of a perceived measure of "difference" or "deviance" from socially prescribed norms of family life, motherhood, and personhood. At this outer edge, one has the experience of radical isolation but also the possibility of a "different" view of the center, a different view of family life, motherhood, and personhood that is both subversive and liberating.

In my experience, mothers of children with disabilities are marginalized largely through being socially invisible, an invisibility that is both part of and distinct from the social invisibility of people with disabilities themselves. We just don't exist. Where are we? And what are we doing?

## A DAY IN THE LIFE

On the good days I compare my life with Esther to dancing on a high wire without a net. It is an exhilarating adventure. I feel fully alive and invigorated. I am focused in the moment, and the view is great. But there is always that edge: If I miss a step will I end up in the pit down below, bruised and hurting?

Esther is up and chattering on about the day ahead of her long before I can manage a coherent sentence. Her 14-year old sister, Anna, a "normal" child, has been independent in the morning for many years, having learned early this part of her adaptation to being Esther's sibling. As of this year, Esther can on most days route herself to the bathroom directly and take off her own pull-up diaper. After 7 years of painstaking and frustrating morning work teaching Esther how to dress herself, she is able to put on her own undershirt, shirt, underpants, pants, and socks—and these garments are mostly faced in the right direction. She sometimes manages her own leg braces, but her shoes require assistance. This year, however, with the addition of a back brace for her scoliosis, her hard-won quasi-independence in dressing herself has been set back. The body brace needs to be centered and carefully put on or it will do her no good. Its purpose is to keep her scoliosis from worsening and to avert a spinal surgery that holds little promise of helping her, because her scoliosis is "functional"—caused by her "chronic hypotonia" or low muscle tone throughout her body, part of a medical and developmental condition without a diagnosis.

Esther is a slow-moving child in a fast-paced world. She must be on her school bus by 7:35 A.M. Even if she were more able-bodied, there is no way she could get ready by herself quickly enough to make the bus unless she got up at the crack of dawn. Having Esther wake up earlier to take the time to be more independent is not a good option because without enough sleep she becomes more vulnerable to illness. Esther gets sick frequently. Last year, she missed more than 65 days of school. What could be a mild cold for most "normal" children turns into a chronic allergic asthmatic cough that can last for as long as 2 or more weeks. On the days Esther stays home, inhaling albuterol from her nebulizer and becoming more and more listless, my life and her father Roger's, become centered around her health care and the tricky balancing act of not neglecting Anna in the process.

After Esther is dressed, she eats her breakfast, leaving a small hill of crumbs at her feet, because her hand use is also affected by her condition. She ingests a daily medicinal armamentarium of supplements, herbs, and drugs to strengthen her immune system and treat her asthma. Our dining room cabinet, the kind usually resplendent with knickknacks and tableware, contains four shelves dedicated to Esther's health. The asthma medication and equipment shelf is laden with sodium chloride inhalation solution, Vanceril, Proventil, Tilade, inhalers. Chinese herbs, homeopathic remedies, blue-green algae, and digestive enzymes occupy the second shelf. The Western herbal tinctures share a shelf with DMSO, a non-FDA approved drug that is prescribed by a physician who has researched this medication for neurological conditions. The bottom shelf holds miscellaneous necessities—handweights, theraputty, and spongy balls to strengthen Esther's hands, arm slings used for broken bones. Esther slugs down vitamins and blue-green algae, drinks her "power drink" and foul-smelling Chinese brew, and inhales her Vanceril without complaining. She's a pro at pill popping and medications.

After an hour of labor by Roger or an hour and a half by me (Roger is a faster helper than I am), Esther is launched to school. Each morning, as she gets on the bus, I silently pray that she will come back in one piece. By 8 years of age, Esther had fractured eight bones. Several of these breaks were from simple falls that most kids would just brush off. She is at risk for these multiple injuries and fractures for reasons that are not well medically understood. *Goddess, I release her into your care, and I pray that you guide and protect her.* My ritual prayer as she gets on the school bus or ventures anywhere out of my sight, helps me let go of the hypervigilance that I have had to exercise in being her mother.

It is usually Roger who picks up Esther after school. He has an academic schedule, while I see clients in the afternoon. One of us accompanies her to a variety of afterschool activities that include vision therapy (for her problems with tracking, focusing, and depth perception), Hebrew school, music therapy, and choir.

Fortunately, Esther receives occupational therapy, physical therapy and speech therapy at school, otherwise there would not be enough hours in the day to take her on her daily and weekly rounds of special-needs care. Or alternatively, it would require that one of her parents take a permanent leave of absence from work, a sometimes inviting but highly impractical possibility. Every several weeks, depending on her state of health, she visits one or more of a dozen health care providers or therapists including pediatrician, orthopedist, asthma and allergy specialist, otolaryngologist, acupuncturist, and chiropractor. Visiting doctors is a permanent way of life for the parents of a child with special needs. In Esther's case, so is the continual search for ways to help her with a condition that has no name. Her mild hearing loss, chronic allergies, sinusitis, asthma, lowered immune system, severe difficulties in the perceptual–motor realm, generalized learning disabilities, foot deformities, hypotonia, poor balance and coordination, and vulnerability to bone fractures are all part of a puzzle that no one seems to be able to fit together. Nor do we know if knowing how it all fits together would be particularly helpful to her or to us. In the meantime, we research ways to help her, and my "Esther" files, which fill a two-drawer file cabinet, continue to grow.

In the evening, one of us helps Esther with her homework, which is done on the computer because her handwriting is minimal. Her nightly bedtime routine includes being helped with her bath and evening medications, being read to, and having her back and feet massaged before she goes to sleep. Esther is usually in pain by the end of the day; the muscles of her back, neck, feet, and legs are tired and sore. The massage is also to help her relax because though exhausted, she often has some trouble turning off her energy and becomes maddeningly perseverative when she's tired. The last words that Esther hears each night are my prayers: *May your healing be complete, may you stand on your own two feet. May I be patient with you, may you be patient with me. May you always be full of life and love and know that you are loved. God bless you and be with you. Now go to sleep.*

\*     \*     \*

I have assistance in raising Esther that far surpasses what mothers of children with disabilities received in other eras or receive now in other societies. I am entitled to $900 annually for "respite care" from the state of Massachusetts, to be spent for a "respite care worker" who gets paid $9.00 per hour. Esther's education in an integrated program in a private school is paid for by the Boston Public School system, thanks to the "766" state law by which each child is entitled to an education in the "least restrictive environment." The synagogue to which we belong pays for an aide in Esther's Hebrew and Religious school classrooms. I live in a city that puts out the excellent *Exceptional Parent Magazine,* which brings me monthly installments of relevant news, information, and support.

Most of all, I am not alone in raising Esther. Roger is as much Esther's "mother" as I am. (She inadvertently still uses "Dad" or "Mom" interchangeably to refer to either one of us.) Coparenting of this kind is the exception, not the rule in the care of most children. This is especially so for children with disabilities, whose parents have a significantly higher rate of divorce than the general population and who are then raised by single mothers. Roger's involvement in Esther's care—and the privilege of his academic schedule, which permits him to spend much more time with Esther than most working fathers could—allows us to break down the labor. Roger does more of the morning and evening daily maintenance, while I am Esther's overall care coordinator. On average, I spend as much time taking Esther to doctors; coordinating her care; and researching educational, therapeutic, and medical resources as I do working in my profession as a psychotherapist, having limited my private practice and consulting to part-time since her birth.

Though Esther has two "mothers," it's still a rare day when either one of us feels adequate to the job. There is always something essential that falls to the ground while we juggle the other six balls. On a bad day, I feel like Sisyphus of the Greek myth. Pushing his huge stone up the mountain, he exerts a prodigious effort to get it to the top. And just as he does, the stone begins to roll down the mountain due to the force of gravity, rolling right over Sisyphus on its unrelenting way down. He must then start all over again—only to confront the same crush, endlessly into the future. Just when things seem to even out, a new set of daunting challenges presents itself. There are times when everything seems to fall apart—when Esther's normal daily needs are complicated by prolonged periods of illness and I am confined to my house, my spirits dimmed by the sound of her asthmatic cough; when I must put the rest of my life "on hold" in order to tend to her; when all sense of order disappears under a pile of unfinished tasks. At these times, I enter a state beyond fatigue that is akin to despair.

Furthermore, the traditional social expectations of motherhood die hard. Most mothers internalize a standard of mother care in which the expectation is that the fundamental responsibility for the care of the child is mother's work. Those of us who cannot afford a live-in nanny or full-time aide, or who do not wish to hand to professionals the total care of our children, still have to grapple with this expectation. This feeds a sense that we are responsible for a job that no single person is capable of doing, which is a recipe for feeling inadequate.

The pain and exhaustion of the hard times has as much to do with how our society throws families in general onto their own individualized and atomized resources—resources often scant enough for the "normal" family and inadequate or catastrophic for the "disabled" family—as it does with Esther's needs. It has as much to do with not being able to afford all of the out-of-network, out-of-pocket health care that she could use as it does with her chronic medical problems. It has as much to do with how poorly our society deals with "otherness" as it does with Esther's "difference." If, as the saying goes, "it takes a village to raise a child," then special-needs children need that village even more than others do. The absence of that village—of community support and of an honest, balanced, informed, communal understanding of the joys, challenges, and difficulties of raising a child with disabilities—not only contributes to what's disabling about disability, but is at the core of what perpetuates a sense of mothering at the margins.

## THE SILENCE OF THE MOTHERS

Many mothers of children with disabilities prefer to keep their pain and exhaustion private, not wanting to fuel the argument that children with disabilities are a "burden" to their parents and to society. This is a self-enforced silencing that is part of what it means to be "marginalized." As I see it, mothers disproportionately shoulder the "burden" precisely because the social marginalization of mothers and of disability are at the heart of what's overwhelming about raising a "different" child.

I recently attended a conference on mothers and daughters at which one of the speakers was a mother of a grown child with multiple physical, cognitive, and developmental disabilities. She spoke about how mothering such a child is in many ways no different than mothering any child. One is called to love and to nurture, to discipline and to guide, to accept and enjoy the child for who she or he is, to lay the fertile ground in which the child's individual gifts can flourish. I was struck by the fact that only in a society in which the intolerance of difference is endemic to our way of thinking is it necessary to make the point that our children, whatever their "special needs," are still children, and that we mothers, whatever our differences from "normal" mothers, are still mothers. Is this "normalization" of difference necessary? Sadly, yes.

I was prompted to add a comment to this speaker's words—that however much we are like "normal" mothers, mothers of children with disabilities also do many things that "normal" mothers don't do and think about many things that "normal" mothers don't think about. Feeding a child through a gastric tube inserted into the stomach; tending to her toileting needs throughout her life; researching the medical literature on a particular diagnosis; managing the complex bureaucracies of special education, medical treatment, and insurance companies, to cite just a few examples, are generally not what mothers envision when we sign on for the job. In my experience, it is rare for mothers of children with disabilities to tell it like it is when it comes to how atypical a typical day in the life can be. In response to my comment, the speaker at this conference admitted that for many years she kept silent about the physical and emotional demands of the daily routines of caring for her daughter, believing that she must bear her lot stoically to be a "good mother."

The pressures of what it takes to be a "good mother" are applied to all mothers, but are particularly isolating when the challenges of being a "good mother" are heightened by disability. I have felt this kind of pressure from school officials or doctors when advocating for Esther and know several mothers who have had similar experiences. Anything less than a serene or stoic attitude to the difficulties of raising our children may be counted as a failure of "good mothering." To speak of the burdens along with the pleasures of mothering may be seen as proof that we are "unresolved" about our children's disabilities, too hyperinvolved and unable to "separate" from them adequately, thus damaging their self-esteem or worsening their disabilities. Silence about the difficulties and necessary sacrifices of raising our children seems to be the requisite of "good mothering."

This is one of the main reasons I include my unadorned chronicle of a day in the life. If my day with Esther sounds laborious and difficult, this doesn't mean that mothering Esther is not also a delight and a gift. But neither does the delight cancel out the difficulties. I think it is important for all mothers to resist silencing, censoring, and "disappearing" ourselves for the sake of holding up the cultural image of "good mothering."

## INVISIBILITY

When Esther was 3 years old, we spent a few weeks at a family meditation retreat in Barre, Massachusetts. Esther had learned to walk 6 months before, a newly born colt. One afternoon I stood with her on the great green lawn, watching as the able-bodied children ran and jumped and tumbled. Someone's daughter, a practiced and near-professional gymnast, was working out on the lawn, doing cartwheels and spins that seemed as effortless as breathing. My awe at the agility of the human body had been heightened by the troubles that Esther has with movement and coordination. I took in this athletic and graceful performance with a mixture of awe and grief, admiration and envy. As I wondered if I would ever be able to look at an able-bodied child again without that particular mix of feelings, the man who stood next to me on the lawn, a practiced meditator in the Vipassana (Insight) meditation tradition, said of the young gymnast spinning a cartwheel before us, "Isn't she just superb? Children are so graceful and agile, aren't they?" I was speechless. I felt in that moment that this man was addressing himself to a ghost, and that I was that ghost, my substantiality not perceivable to him. This young girl was most certainly superb, graceful, and agile. But his use of the universalizing plural noun, the absoluteness of his exclamation that "children are so graceful," addressed to me as my Esther, barely able to stand without falling and as easily blown over as a leaf in the wind, stood in plain sight before us, made it clear that this man, trained in awareness, was simply not *seeing* Esther. She was as invisible to him as I was. He saw only the gymnast and, from this partial sight, spun his tales about children.

The generation of children born to the baby boomers is in fact the most visible generation of children with disabilities in the industrial West. Handicap accessibility has arrived on the scene in the past two decades. We now see people going about their business in wheelchairs in ways that were once impossible. As recently as 20 years ago, mothers of children with Down syndrome or other birth defects were routinely advised on their birthbeds to institutionalize their "defective" offspring. We see "different" children in public in greater numbers than ever before. "Sped" or special education is an expected part of most public school systems. Massachusetts has a law guaranteeing the right to an education in the "least restrictive environment" to every child with special needs, and other states have comparable laws. Still, our senses can close themselves off to whatever we do not wish to see. And this closing off on the part of the able-bodied keeps both child and mother on the periphery of consciousness, the outside edge of everything we call "normal" life. We are generally educated in our society to not see the disabled and their families, who appear to be a blot on the very idea of the "normal" family and of "normal" life itself.

## MOTHERING A "DIFFERENT" CHILD IN A "NORMAL" WORLD

Crippled. Disabled. Handicapped. Child with disabilities. Special-needs child. Physically challenged. Differently abled. Developmentally delayed. I don't like any of these words. They are either stigmatizing and limiting (crippled, disabled, handicapped), thereby contributing to the person's "disability," or they are patronizingly euphemistic (physically challenged, developmentally delayed), a reaction to the stigmatizing and limiting words. Or they are just "politically correct" but largely useless (differently abled). Our language has no way to express the condition of someone who has physical, mental or educational needs that are more than what is typical of others, without invoking a standard of normalcy or patronizingly avoiding it. It has no way of describing a condition that requires the help of others in a respectful and not paternalistic way.

One day I was rushing the kids to the dinner table and my oldest daughter Anna wasn't sure she wanted to eat with us at that hour. To her question "Why do I have to eat dinner when you do?" my quick and unthoughtful answer was "Because I enjoy eating dinner like a normal family." Without missing a beat, Anna exclaimed, "Mom, there's no such thing as normal!" "You're absolutely right," I said, grateful for how Anna always catches me up in my thoughtless replies. "I want you at dinner," I corrected myself, "because I enjoy your company."

A sign in my private practice psychotherapy office reads "Why be normal?" Growing up, I never much took to the idea of normalcy. As an adolescent, I remember praying, like the girl in the play *The Fantasticks,* "Please, God, don't let me be normal." With a child's-eye view of the world that came from being the daughter of Holocaust survivors, I did not find the measure of the "normal" a comforting one. From an early age, it seemed to me that normal people had committed all the small, daily, ordinary, and extraordinary acts that became, when all was said and done, the Holocaust. And that normal people had let it happen. I didn't want to be that kind of normal.

The problem lies in our culture's entire way of categorizing people into normal and abnormal, mainstream and deviant. We can't even imagine what it would be like to think outside of this dominant dichotomy and its inherent ideology of difference. Who are the normal? And who the different? In our culture, the norm for normal is the white male without any *visible* physical or mental deficits. The "normal" male is the standard-bearer for qualities that are highly valued in the culture, such as independence. But judged against a standard derived from the margin, for instance, a more female norm of human empathy, the "normal" (male) person seems rather deficient. The difference between normal and deviant depends on where you stick the sign that says "normal starts here." Philosophically, morally, and practically, the fundamental idea of "normal" is troublesome, erecting a hierarchy that inherently reproduces a false sense of competence or a debilitating sense of shame in those who fall into the normal or abnormal categories, respectively. The fundamental ideology of normalcy–deviance by which that which is "normal" stands in sharp contrast to that which is "different"—and which contrast constitutes an a priori devaluation of the latter—is nowhere more virulent and destructive than it is with respect to people with visible disabilities. There is no disability, however genetically or biochemically based, that is not profoundly worsened by the way we marginalize, stigmatize, and refuse to recognize people who are visibly different from this hypothetical norm. Some in the disability rights movement would say that disability is itself constructed, that what we see as individual disability is as much a product of the social marginalization of "defectives" as it is of the particular "defect." And that the disability itself would actually look and function differently, would be less disabling, if we had a less disabled and disabling society.

Standards of normalcy affect the very way that we think about what it means to be a person, and the way that we feel about a person's inherent worth. We think of certain lives as "worth living" and others as less so or not at all. Hitler brought this way of thinking to its fascist extreme in his program of eugenics and euthanasia by which the sick, "deformed," and "defective" were cleansed from society for the sake of Aryan health. Mental and physical "defectives" were first on Hitler's list of "useless eaters"—before homosexuals and Jews. At the Auschwitz museum, the prostheses of these "defectives" are exhibited in piles, along with the piles of shoes, hair, and eyeglasses taken from the Jews. Many who would look in horror at these displays of Nazi hatred may still share in some way the idea that certain lives are less valuable than others. On this basis, they may make decisions about having an abortion, for instance, or about whether to fund the medical needs of a Down syndrome baby as opposed to a "normal" one.

These questions of normalcy and difference are complex and fraught with moral, philosophical, and practical dilemmas and ambiguities. But the way that they affect me as the mother of a child who is not "normal" is quite simple. The shame of the "not normal" is a condition that one must continually refuse to carry. And refusing to do so makes every day an opportunity for resistance. Accompanying Esther to a new classroom, taking a walk with her in the arboretum, taking her to a play, these everyday occurrences sometimes result in contact with people who blind themselves to Esther's disabilities out of ignorance or fear, or who gape unabashedly at her in a way that they would not do with a "normal" person. Shame easily comes with this territory. Sometimes the staring stems from simple curiosity, which is why I always prefer, as does Esther, to have her special difficulties and needs openly known rather than hidden from others. On the other hand, I have seen children back away from Esther, refuse to sit next to her, stare in a hostile fashion, or shun her as though the shame of her condition might rub off on them. In some instances, Esther is oblivious to this, probably because she doesn't understand social cues as well as she might or because of her perceptual difficulties. The more she becomes aware of her otherness, the more she talks to me about feeling bad. We have talked frequently about how some kids tease or ignore other kids as a way of trying to feel better about themselves, or because they are ignorant. She has heard me say, "No matter what someone may say or do, never forget that no one is better than you." She has also heard me repeat, "You're very good at doing hard things—and that's something many others, to whom things come more easily, are not so good at," and "Whatever you can or can't do, you are a generous, loving, wise person, and nothing is more important than that." In reminding Esther of her worth, I find a way to lift the mantle of shame that can fall so swiftly and silently on the shoulders of one who sees her child treated as "other." The shame of the "not normal" is ultimately the shame that our culture must bear for its intolerance and fear of "difference." I remember a funny song Anna made up years ago, with the refrain "We're all the same in a special way," incorporating the resistance that Anna is learning as Esther's thoughtful older sister. I wish the "normal" world could learn this song's simple truth.

## MARGINALIZING MYTHS

The ideology of normalcy–deviance goes along with a number of related social mythologies that have an impact on the lives of mothers of children with disabilities: the myths of meritocracy and of IQ, the myth of the moral virtue of physical excellence, and, last but not least, the grand American myth of individualism and independence. All of these are operative in my life with Esther.

### Meritocracy and IQ

The myth of meritocracy tells us that what gets rewarded in our society is hard work and merit. There is no one I know who works harder than Esther at simply getting through a day. The sheer effort of holding herself upright, of keeping her eyes focused, her muscles working, her mind attentive when there are so many obstacles in the way of her obvious intelligence, this is not the sort of thing that is or ever will be rewarded in a society that prides itself on rewarding hard work and merit—and that generally rewards those born to a certain class, race, or gender privilege. How do we define "merit?" In our society, merit is synonymous with achievement. We call a life of achievement a "successful" life. And merit-as-achievement is measured by how much status, power, and money it commands. The merit in Esther's life is clear and moving to anyone who knows her, but it cannot be measured in this way. Knowing Esther is, in many ways, like living with a human barometer of our society's illusions about itself.

I don't expect that Esther will go to Harvard. Still, I marvel at what she knows. When she was 5 years old, we watched a TV show together in which a father who had a poor relationship with his daughter became verbally abusive to her. "He's mad because he's sad," Esther informed me. I had certainly not told her this, although as a therapist I know that a lot of rage stems from intolerable sorrow. I thought about what the world would look like, how much more liveable and less violent it would be, if the Esthers of the world were viewed as teachers of emotional intelligence. By first grade, Esther was emotionally adept in ways that are not so much precocious as extraordinary in a society that is just beginning to understand the meaning of the term "emotional intelligence." One evening as she took her bath, I was in a state of emotional turmoil about a relationship with a friend that was disintegrating. I thought I was hiding it very well, being as upbeat as I could while Esther played with her rubber duckie. "What's wrong, Mom?" she wanted to know. "You're feeling sad?" For the next 20 minutes, she asked me a series of pointed questions about this relationship and our emotions about it, ending with a suggestion that I write my friend a letter after we'd each cooled down our anger. She was thinking about how we could reconcile our differences. Though her educational record said that she had problems with attention span, they were certainly not evident in this conversation. A tape of our talk would be a great teaching tool for training new psych interns in listening skills.

When my husband's father was dying, our family arrived just in time to sit by his bedside and be with him for the last half hour of his life. Esther was 6 years old. She sat quietly and looked at the old man's face very closely. Some months later, she asked Roger if he was sad about his father's death. When Roger answered that he was, Esther said, "I know how you feel. But it was his time to die. And it's good that you got there before he died so he was able to hear you say the shema [the central prayer in Judaism]." At times when the family has been in crisis or emotional difficulty (often the crisis is a medical emergency involving Esther's health), she is prone to saying things like "Let's say thank you for what we have." Esther could find the bright side of the moon on the darkest night. Her wisdom is inexhaustible and has seen her, and us, through many such nights. It is not that Esther is learning her spiritual wisdom from us; she is not the student but the teacher in this realm. I am her student, a slow learner with a host of developmental delays.

Still, by the calculations of intelligence applied in the rationalist, positivist, number-crunching world in which we live, Esther's special intelligence is incalculable, and it is therefore invisible. The concept of IQ as a number roughly equivalent to a culture-bound test of one's mathematical and verbal agility, and tested by a standardized multiple-choice format, comes crashing down on Esther's future. Will people in her future be able to see beyond her "handicaps" to who she really is? The quality of her life will depend in large measure on the answer to this question. Will our society develop the intelligence to break through its own myth of IQ? Only if it is willing to learn from its children with "learning disabilities" and "mental retardation." Perhaps the children of this generation of baby boomers—the first in history to advocate strongly and passionately for the public inclusion of their children in all walks of life—will be instrumental in bringing the wisdom of our children to the world.

### Physical Excellence as Moral Virtue

The myth of physical excellence as the apex of virtue and value is in evidence more and more in our society. There are aerobics classes in every gym and Y, every health and fitness center. Getting fit is not only good for you, it shows you are better than those poor slobs who don't have the inclination, time, or able-bodiedness to engage in the Workout. Whom do we most worship in this society and make our household icons, like gods of yore? Movie stars and sports players. The beautiful and the athletic. We pay these icons outrageous and obscene amounts of money, heaping fame and fortune on them for their superior gifts. Muhammad Ali, the former Cassius Clay, is the most known figure in the world. Michael Jordan is treated as a hero for his ability to throw a ball into a hoop. Those who exhibit athletic excellence are the ones we make our cultural heroes. If we rewarded those who show fortitude in the face of adversity with the same kind of fame and fortune that we heap on those who take a gymnastic leap on a sprained ankle, we would have a world more hospitable to human life. Esther would be rich, my life would be a lot easier, and I'm sure I'd be a less stressed-out, better mother.

## Independence and Individualism

Perhaps the bedrock ideology that affects my everyday life as a mother is the myth of independent individualism. Through this myth we elevate a standard of autonomy that is, on close inspection, a denial of our fundamental interdependence as human beings. "No man (woman, or child) is an island." Those we credit with this rock-like independence tend to be those whose dependence is generally unacknowledged or hidden, including the dependence of the entrepreneur on the worker, the working father on the stay-at-home mother. The hidden dependencies that we revile and castigate, disavow or shun in ourselves, we find hard to take in those whose needs for help are out there and visible every minute. This is one reason why we ghettoize and institutionalize those who are visibly different and "needy." We can't stand looking at them. They remind us that we too are vulnerable; that we are dependent on others; that we have needs, which we consider, in the dominant masculine ideology of our society, to be shameful weaknesses without merit.

One of the first phrases Esther learned to say was "I need help." She still says it often and without shame. What in the world would change, I wonder, if instead of encouraging the Esthers of the world to internalize the dominant norms of independent individualism, our society were to learn from these "different" children how to speak up without shame about the human need for each other's help? What if we developed egos built around the simple reality of interdependence? My sense of living at the margins would in all likelihood disappear. And perhaps we'd all be able, at last, to let go of our obsessions about who's better than whom, and rejoice, as Esther does, in simply being together.

## MEDICAL MARGINALIZATION

In one of the support groups I attended years ago for parents of children with disabilities, we compiled a list of topics we wanted to discuss. At the top of the list was "doctors." Nobody had to ask why we needed to share our doctor stories. We were all veterans of the medical system, each with our own bag of medical horror stories and advocacy triumphs. I remember one mother of a child with severe cerebral palsy who said, "The worst part of being Adam's mother is having to see doctors all the time. They know so much less than they think, and they do as much damage as good." Her words were stark but, I think, descriptive of the experience of many mothers of special-needs children. Esther has seen a total of more than 200 helpers, healers, doctors, and therapists in the decade of her life. From faith healer to neurologist, from allergist to physiatrist (a specialty we knew nothing about and that proved to be absolutely useless). Special-needs children are highly medicalized people, and this medicalization is one of the primary causes of the marginalization of mothers. For the most part, it is mothers who take their children to doctors and who must confront the challenges and limitations of the medical system in relation to a child who is dependent on the system.

Esther's first pediatrician was a man with a gold-star reputation and Harvard credentials, a man who teaches pediatric residents how to be physicians. From the moment of Esther's birth, I knew this baby was in trouble, though her Apgar scores (which rate a newborn's physical condition) were fine and there were no obvious medical problems. From my experience breastfeeding Anna, it was clear to me that Esther was not able to latch onto the breast properly, and that when she did, she easily disengaged. My pediatrician treated my concerns as the excessive preoccupations of a worried mother. He therefore ignored them until they became life threatening. I had to march into his office and insist that he examine the baby. She was seriously dehydrated; he told me to put her on the bottle and threatened to hospitalize her if she didn't gain a substantial amount of weight in 24 hours. He never acknowledged in any way that his inability to respond to my concerns had put her in jeopardy. It is not at all unusual for doctors to ignore the intuitions and insights of mothers, but when dealing with children with special needs, this can lead to serious and even fatal consequences. In addition, the mother's sense of adequacy and ability to protect her child is assaulted.

Esther's second pediatrician, named one of "Boston's Best," shrugged his shoulders soulfully whenever he was asked if he knew of anything that might help with Esther's development. "Let's just wait and see" was his mantra, which was a recipe for disaster with a child like Esther. All of her early therapies—speech, occupational, and physical—were arranged by me with barely a nod of interest from him.

In the 2 years he was Esther's doctor, her health deteriorated. She was continuously ill with coughs that kept her, and us, up at night. Each time she became ill, his diagnosis was the same. "It's a virus," he would say, and he would prescribe antibiotics when it didn't disappear after 2 weeks. A week after the antibiotic was finished, she would be sick again. I knew that something else was amiss with Esther's health and requested a consultation. Desperate from sleep deprivation and worry, I had been reading pediatric medical books on respiratory illnesses. I believed that Esther might have asthma or perhaps even whooping cough, for which she had not been innoculated because the neuromotor nature of her disability put her at risk for serious side effects of the pertussis vaccine. The doctor listened, barely able to contain his impatience. "I can take care of your child," he said, "but I cannot take care of you." Fighting back tears, I told him that communicating about Esther's recurrent illnesses was part of his role as her physician, and that if he chose to see this as my need to be "taken care of," then indeed I wanted him to respond to this need. If he didn't see this as his job, then perhaps he should not be Esther's pediatrician. I left shaken and distraught.

Two days later, the doctor telephoned. "You are right, and I was wrong," he said. "I'll try to do better." I was enormously relieved. He did finally refer Esther to a pulmonary specialist, who said she had either asthma or whooping cough and with the latter test being negative, diagnosed the asthma that had been plaguing her and us for more than a year. There was some relief once she was on medication. But the fact is, even with his best intentions and his admirable ability to apologize, this doctor continued to pay inadequate attention to Esther's medical needs, and I ended up leaving his practice some months later.

A physician's inability to handle his own emotions about disability—or about the struggle and persistence of mothers of children with disabilities—can lead to a host of problems. Some doctors don't want a mother as "co-equal" in the treatment of the child and are put off by mothers who have learned, of necessity how to advocate strongly for their children. Others can't cope with the helplessness they feel in the face of many chronic disabilities. Trained to "cure," doctors of special-needs children are often confronted with situations in which no cure is available and/or treatment is risky or offers little. Because Esther has no known diagnosis, there is a sense of chronic uncertainty that is emotionally difficult for doctors as well as parents. The problem is that the cult of the medical expert produces physicians who are often less than forthright about the limits of their knowledge or procedures. They tend to make one of two mistakes: Either they do something when there is nothing to be done, largely as a way of treating their own feelings of helplessness, which may result in a plethora of unnecessary and even damaging procedures or surgeries, or they do nothing when they should do something. The latter mistake comes mostly from doctors who don't know how to listen to mothers, patronizing us when they should be paying respectful and close attention to what we know.

Emotions like sorrow, frustration, and fear come with the territory of being a mother of a special-needs child. But medical culture promotes an intolerance of emotions in the treatment situation where they are most likely to be present, that is, medical crises. This is a recipe for the unwitting and pervasive marginalization of mothers by the very doctors on whom we depend to help our children. The result is not only an additional burden of pain for the mother but an impoverished practice of medicine.

## MARGINALIZATION IN EDUCATION

Esther attends a school with an "integrated" program for children with differing needs. The Boston public school system pays for this because, by state law, every child is entitled to be educated in the "least restrictive environment." It took 6 months of intensive labor to advocate for and get this placement for Esther—a process that involved researching schools, researching the law, getting Esther evaluated, hiring a lawyer, and then facing down Court Street, the headquarters of the Boston school system. The evaluation process consisted of a 5-minute observation of Esther at play and a routine psychological exam that ignored her physical disabilities. On this basis, it was recommended that Esther be placed in a segregated kindergarten classroom in which she would be the only child who was not mentally retarded. When Roger and I successfully fought this, the next recommendation was one of the handful of integrated classrooms in the Boston school system at the time. It was a lovely school—but both inacessible and unsafe for Esther. The director of the school had not been informed of the extent of Esther's physical limitations. Yet I was advised by my attorney that talking to the director myself would hurt my case, and that I should resort to an arduous and expensive court battle instead. I chose to go against his advice and took Esther to meet the director face to face. Fifteen minutes later, the director declared, "Esther would not be safe here." Boston then consented to the school of our choice. It was a victory, but one that could have been accomplished with far less wear and tear on all parties if it were not for the routine marginalization of mothers by both attorneys and school bureaucracies.

The private sector can claim no moral highground here. Unlike public schools, private schools are not mandated by law to admit any children with special needs. In my experience, the private school priority of quality education for the "whole child" leaves children like Esther outside the door. For a time, I considered sending Esther to the private school that Anna attended. I spent 2 years on the "diversity committee" at this school, trying to prepare the way for Esther's entrance to kindergarten. I was treated with polite aloofness. People "forgot" to tell me when the next meeting was. The head of the school suggested a study of the school's "capability" for inclusion—a study that was never done. In the last meeting I attended, a father on the committee looked me straight in the eye and said: "There's no place for a child like yours at this school. It would cost too much." I appreciated his honesty. The word "diversity" simply didn't apply to Esther in this "progressive" private school setting.

When Anna, then age 7, asked one day if Esther would be going to her school and learned that I was considering it, she became alarmed. "No!" she cried, "I don't want her to go." Asked why, she answered, "Because she wouldn't be safe in the yard. And because the school doesn't want her." Startled, I wanted to know what made her think so. She answered with the impeccable logic of the child who saw the nakedness of the emperor in *The Emperor's New Clothes*: "Because there's nobody like her at the school. If they wanted kids like her there, they would have them."

Resistance to marginalization in education has everything to do with mothers becoming hard-nosed advocates for our children while not becoming unduly adversarial. Of necessity, I have honed my skills in this area and I know they will stand me in good stead for Esther's forseeable future.

## MARGINALIZATION
## FROM OTHER MOTHERS

Recently, I heard Michael Berube read from his book about parenting a Down syndrome child. After the reading, a woman in the audience raised her hand. About 60 years old, she talked about her grown son, whom she called "slow." "When he was in elementary school the children were all right with my son, but the mothers weren't," she said. "So my son had no friends, because none of the mothers wanted him at their house. It was as though he had a contagious disease." The pain in this elderly mother's voice was still fresh, after all the years. And many in the audience, also parents of special needs children, nodded knowingly or wiped tears from their faces.

The psychological and social roots of the marginalization of mothers of disabled children interract and reinforce one another. In the context of the American cultural ideal of an easy, comfortable life, visible adversity can appear unvirtuous, a sign of personal failure. The resultant shame for those who suffer misfortune is complicated and worsened by the ways that many people distance themselves from a life of noticeable pain. This distancing is not always intentional or even conscious. It is difficult to see the vulnerability of special-needs families without feeling some trace of fear, helplessness, or guilt—emotions that can push people out of connection when these feelings are not recognized or cannot be an open, spoken aspect of relationship. Ours is what I call an emotion-phobic culture. It has a low threshold of tolerance for uncomfortable or painful emotions like guilt, fear, sorrow, or helplessness and discourages the disclosure of such feelings. When we marginalize "negative" emotions, it is easy to marginalize the people who trigger them. The human tendency to seek pleasure and avoid pain makes marginalization of mothers of disabled children predictable. What makes it worse is the American preoccupation with the easy life and our culture's emotional illiteracy.

Marginalization hurts, but the isolation of difference is not written in the stars. It is emotionally, socially, and economically constructed. I have met parents of special-needs children who deal with their sense of isolation by surrounding themselves exclusively with other special-needs families. This self-imposed ghettoization is a course I have not chosen because I believe it is simply isolation in another form. On the other hand, there are those families who try to "pass" by essentially hiding their children's disabilities, where possible, and keeping their struggles a secret. This form of denial takes a serious toll on both child and family. I have tried to steer a course between being totally identified as "mother of disabled child" and living in the denial zone. I think of this course as a form of resistance to the cultural imposition of the normal–abnormal line that, like the color line, keeps everyone in their place and keeps us from touching one another's lives. I am delighted that Esther was the first child with a disability to "integrate" the Farm and Wilderness Day Camp in Vermont, ushering in a new era in which children with Down syndrome and cerebral palsy now get to enjoy the wonders of nature hikes and sleeping out under the stars, along with their able-bodied friends.

## SPIRITUAL RESISTANCE

Mothering Esther is about parenting without a developmental map. This is in some sense true for all mothers because every child is unique, but for me, there are none of the usual reassurances of "normal" one-size-fits-all parenting and one-size-fits-all models of child development. There is a freedom that comes with this kind of marginalization. The questions about Esther's future hang uncertainly in the air: Will she or won't she have the same needs and disabilities tomorrow as she has today? How many of them will improve? How many remain? Will she be able to live independently? With what kind of help? None of us really know how our children will end up, but we may surround ourselves with illusions of safety and certainty. In mothering Esther, not knowing is the name of the game. It teaches the spiritual discipline of living in the present moment while planning for a future that is, by definition, uncertain. There are days when this challenge brings nothing but anxiety. But as a whole, I believe it has been a profound teacher of spiritual steadfastness and courage. It is Esther herself who is my role model here, teaching me to experience my life with her and my family as a challenging adventure.

\*     \*     \*

Our family is vacationing in Vermont. Esther is the first child with disabilities at the Farm and Wilderness Barn Day Camp. She is 6 years old and determined to ride a bike. Roger and I rig up a souped-up tricycle that we think will be safe for her. We take turns teaching her. Anna, eager for Esther to learn, spends some time teaching her as well. It seems Esther has the essentials down. There is a moment where I take a deep breath and turn indoors to cook dinner.

I let go of my eternal mother's vigilance. For once I treat Esther like a "normal" child, and with just a moment's hesitation I simply leave her on the bike. Roger and Anna are at her side. Two minutes later I hear her wail. I run out just in time to see Esther spill off the bike. She soon stops crying and wants to get back on. I look at her hand and help her on, but then see that she seems to be in mild shock. Is her arm broken?

Later, as we sit and eat dinner, Esther says quietly, "I can't use this hand." An X-ray at the local Vermont hospital confirms the fracture in her wrist. It is the fourth fracture in 6 years. At the hospital, Esther is her usual brave and friendly self. She is cheering us up. She is complimenting the doctor on what a good job he is doing putting a cast on her arm. Later she asks him if she can swim. When she is told she cannot swim with the cast on—and that means for the rest of the camp season—she pauses for a second, then says, "That's OK, I'll stay down by the waterfront and put my legs in the water, or I'll go up to the barn with the counselors and sing." Esther loves swimming more than anything in the world except for maybe ice cream and pizza. It is one of the only things she can do where she doesn't look weird and her body is relieved of the constant pull of gravity. How can she be so accepting? She only wants to be included, and finding a way to include herself at the camp, even with her broken wrist, she is happy.

The next morning, she eats breakfast with her good arm and sings a little made-up song that goes, "When you open up your love, love will come to you." She soothes her hand, calling it "beauty star" and sings lullabies to it to make it feel better. Later on, she laughs, "It's just a broken hand. Ha!" Esther teaches me how to mother her. And she is an exceptionally good teacher because just as her muscle tone, her cognition, and her neuromotor system are not "normal," so it is with her ego. She is a little buddha who finds something to be grateful for in the present moment and enjoys it, continually teaching me about love without conditions, care without ownership, the sacred in the broken.

Still, I cannot make her the wisdom child. She has her own struggles and pain. She has no close friends her own age. She is sometimes lonely. She is too attached to TV, her dependable pal. She gets frustrated and perseverates. And I get frustrated, weary, and angry. I pray to be worthy of her. Like dancing on the high wire without a net, I have to let her try, to let her risk, to let her be frustrated and uncomfortable, in order for her to develop new skills. But each time I take a breath and wonder if she'll survive. I know I can't protect her, I can only fight for her and then let her go. I try to remember, where there is fear there is power. And when I do, I can be a source of healing energy for her and she for me.

Esther herself is the best source of whatever courage and resistance I muster in the challenge of mothering her. She has taught me acceptance and gratitude for each moment in a way that has brought a very special kind of joy into my life. She has helped free me of the shackles of a driven achievement orientation to life that comes from my early family training, and the entire culture's premium on performance and obsession with "success." Esther teaches me the absolute value of life, a value that has nothing to do with what she can give me by way of reflecting back my own ego. I am rarely proud of her in the "normal parent" way in which parents narcissistically take credit for their children's accomplishments. When she sings her heart out at a music recital, it is not her near-perfect pitch that I take pride in. What I feel is a sense of awe and gratitude for the amazing beauty of her spirit and the way that it comes through her in song, warming the hearts of those who hear. Everything that Esther is, she has made herself—against tremendous odds. It is not "pride" I feel but genuine respect for who she is as a person. The flip side of Esther's special needs are her special gifts: open-hearted generosity of spirit, compassion, emotional wisdom, and joy in the midst of limitation.

When I told a relative some time ago that Esther's disabilities would be ongoing, that she would not grow out of them as we, her doctors, and teachers had once hoped, he referred to Esther as "the worst nightmare a parent can have." I understood this as his way of trying to be empathetic, though he could only imagine a life of "non-normal" parenting as a nightmare, not as a gift. Actually, I could think of many things I would consider parental "nightmares": murdered children, children with AIDS, teens dying in car crashes, adult children who are battered by boyfriends or raped, children who grow up and work for the Pentagon. As she is, without the comparisons to "normal" by which her life appears to some to be a nightmare, Esther is a continual source of delight and spiritual sustenance in my life. I am blessed to be her mother. Given a choice, I would not choose her to be other than she is, though like all mothers who love their children, I would want her to have a life of good health. If there is a nightmare here, it is my fear that the world, when I leave it, will not be sufficient to hold her or to see her truly. The unanswered question is: Will her gifts find their place in a world not yet worthy of her, or of any of our children?

## BIBLIOGRAPHY

Berube, M. (1996). *Life as we know it: A father, a family, and an exceptional child.* New York: Pantheon Books.

Callahan, M. (1987). *Fighting for Tony.* New York: Simon & Schuster.

Deford, F. (1983). *Alex: The life of a child.* New York: Signet.

Featherstone, H. (1981). *A difference in the family.* New York: Penguin.

Greenfield, J. (1970). *A child called Noah: A family journey.* New York: Harcourt Brace Jovanovich.

Kaufman, B. (1981). *A miracle to believe in.* New York: Fawcett Crest.

Kramer, L. S. (1996). *Uncommon voyage: Parenting a special needs child in the world of alternative medicine.* Boston: Faber and Faber.

Saxton, M., & Howe. F. (1987). *With wings: An anthology of literature by and about women with disabilities.* New York: Feminist Press.

Sienkiewicz-Mercer, R., & Kaplan, S. (1989). *I raise my eyes to say yes.* New York: Avon.

Simons, R. (1987). *After the tears: Parents talk about raising a child with a disability.* New York: Harcourt Brace Jovanovich.

Wendell, S. (1996). *The rejected body: Feminist philosophical reflections on disability.* New York: Routledge.

Wilkinson, S., & Kitzinger, C. (Eds.). (1996). *Representing the other: A feminism and psychology reader.* London: Sage.

# 3

## Homeless
### Mothering at Rock Bottom

REBECCA KOCH
MARY T. LEWIS
WENDY QUIÑONES

SEVEN of us, mothers all, sit together around an office table on a misty winter day. The three "professionals" and authors of this chapter have invited the four others to discuss an area of their expertise: being a mother while being homeless. We are all currently housed, and we all have current or past associations with the same organization, Well spring House, Inc., which has offered us, in different combinations, in different amounts, and at different times, shelter, education, employment, and support.

Wellspring is a nonprofit organization that, among other activities, maintains a small family shelter in a 17th-century home in Gloucester, Massachusetts. Wellspring is a faith community—although not a traditionally religious one—that bases its philosophy and actions on the need for social change rather than social service. Two of us (Lewis and Quiñones) are currently employed there, and one (Koch) is a former employee; the mothers we are talking with have been in shelter there.

In this room, we have already talked about what it means to be a mother. Now two words confront us, written large on newsprint: "homeless mother." What do they mean? From the women who have lived that experience, the responses are immediate and telling:

"Degraded."

"Low-life."

"Shame."

"Out of control."

"Like a failure if you don't have a home for your kids."

"You don't care about your kids enough to give them a nice place."

"It's your decision, because you really could go out and work and do everything. And you can't do everything."

"People definitely think we're not good mothers—just for the fact that we're homeless, we're not good mothers."

"That you somehow quit. That you should have stuck it out, you know? Whatever situation, you should have stuck it out, you shouldn't have ended up here."

"We're burdening the community. All the taxpayers. . . . "

"The taxpayers, oh, yeah, yeah! You can't have anything if you're homeless. God forbid you should have anything if you're homeless, like a car."

"Or a job!"

"I'll never forget when the welfare lady asked me if I had life insurance on my children. I said no, but I asked why. And she said because if you have life insurance, they look at it as income. I said, 'How's that? The kid has to be dead for me to get the money.' She said, 'Well, you know, some people. . . . ' Like excuse me, I'm going to go kill my kid for the money!?"

These voices, these stories, these feelings represent the many others we have heard from homeless mothers through the years. Most have been driven out of their homes by desperate economic circumstances juggled until there are simply too many balls to keep in the air. Some have been dependent for shelter on the goodwill of friends and family until that goodwill is utterly exhausted. Some have suffered and denied physical or sexual abuse of themselves or their children until escape is the only option. Permeating all of their stories is the stink of blame from a society that views poor mothers and their poverty with suspicion and fear. We were familiar with the attitudes about and circumstances of homelessness. But as we examined how motherhood influences becoming homeless, and how being homeless affects mothering, our understanding of our work and its context changed profoundly. This chapter presents some preliminary attempts to reconceptualize both past and ongoing experience. It is an effort to look through a new lens as we examine what is and isn't working in our relationships with homeless mothers. Our conversation is far from being completed, but even this relatively brief exposure to placing mothering at the center of our framework has demonstrated to us the importance of doing so.

## POVERTY, HOMELESSNESS, MOTHERHOOD

"Most people think you bring it all on yourself. I've heard that: 'You brought it all on yourself, you have different choices.' "

Why are people homeless? Because they are too poor to afford homes. Between 1970 and 1995, the number of poor Americans rose from 25.4 million to 36.4 million. Over roughly the same period—from 1973 to 1993—the supply of "affordable" apartments (those that cost no more than 30% of a renter's income) dwindled to produce a shortfall of 4.7 million units, the largest such deficit on record. Other available rentals are simply out of reach, for "in no state does a full-time minimum wage job cover the costs of a one-bedroom unit at fair market rent, and in 45 states and the District of Columbia, families would need to earn at least double the minimum wage in order to afford a two-bedroom unit."[1] Only 26% of households eligible for housing assistance receive it; most housing authorities have waiting lists that are years long. In one 1995 survey of 29 cities, for example, the average wait for various subsidized housing programs ranged from 19 to 32 months. For public housing, waiting lists were 7 years in Chicago, nearly 4 years in Alexandria, Virginia, 3 years in Detroit and Seattle.[2]

"Being homeless affects how I see myself as a mother. Well, if I did the right thing, I wouldn't be here."

[1] Information in the previous two sentences comes from National Coalition for the Homeless (1996).

[2] Information in the previous three sentences comes from U.S. Conference of Mayors (1996).

We are speaking, however, not merely of homeless wage earners, but of homeless mothers who may be or want to be wage earners as well. Mothers and their families are nearly 40% of the homeless in America, a growth of 10% since 1985 and a larger proportion than at any time since the Great Depression (Bassuk, Browne, & Buckner, 1996). It speaks volumes to note that in the 1930s, the response to homelessness was the Social Security Act of 1933, including the first national system of welfare benefits. Today, the response is cuts in those same benefits.

### Homeless Mothers

Who are homeless mothers? Few comprehensive studies exist. But according to recently published findings from an ongoing study of homeless and "poor-housed" mothers in Worcester, Massachusetts, their median age is 27, they have on average two children who are likely to be infants or preschoolers, and they are unlikely to have graduated from high school (Bassuk et al., 1996). Their annual income is likely to be under $7,000, or about half the roughly $13,000 the federal government defines as poverty for a family of three. Massachusetts estimated a family needed $7,081 for rent and utility costs alone in 1995 (Bassuk et al., 1996).

"I was undeserving. I did something to be punished for, because I made a bunch of wrong choices, loved the wrong guy."

Why are homeless mothers so poor? The increasing income disparity in the United States certainly plays a part: In 1993, the top fifth of Americans shared almost half the national income, while those in the bottom fifth competed for only 3.6%.[3] Wage rates diverge by education; in 1993, workers with a full college education earned nearly five times the wages of those who had not completed high school. Gender differences also play a role: Men without high school diplomas earn 58% more than women with a similar education. Illness also compromises earning power, and poor women suffer far more than other women from chronic medical conditions such as asthma, anemia, bronchitis, and ulcers. A final factor is the overriding fact that American mothers—especially single mothers—can count on little or no recognition of their special needs as mothers. This is virtually unique

[3]All statistics in this paragraph are drawn from Bassuk et al. (1996).

among industrialized nations. A single mother of very young children obviously cannot work outside her home unless her children are cared for by someone else. In 1995, 79% of the homeless families in 29 major American cities were headed by a single parent (U.S. Conference of Mayors, 1996), and in the Better Homes Fund study, 59% of women said the unavailability of childcare was a barrier to work (Bassuk et al., 1996). Yet American mothers have access to neither a national system of free childcare, like the French, nor an adequate network of affordable or subsidized care. So the single mother's choices are limited. If she works, she will spend a good proportion of her wages on childcare (in 1993 women earning less than $1,500 per month spent fully 25% of it on child care; Bassuk et al., 1996), or she can stay at home with her children, existing on a level of public support that leaves her with a predictable budget deficit. Under Massachusetts' welfare reform, she may count on even that level of support for only 2 years; the national standard is now no more than 5 years. In either case, she may well end up confronting a painful choice: Will her children have food, or will they have a roof over their heads? She is unlikely to be able to provide both.

## Wellspring's Guests

In 1991, Wellspring conducted research among its former shelter guests, locating and interviewing 79 of the over 200 sheltered to that date. Differing significantly from other samples, Wellspring's former guests were overwhelmingly white (97%) and reasonably well educated (72% had high school diplomas or GEDs, 26% had some college). Like the other groups, however, over three-quarters had two or fewer children; 82% had preschoolers, while fully 50% had children two and younger.

"I have to say, everybody's door is open until they realize that you're going to be there 3, 4 months."

Universally, homelessness among former Wellspring guests was because they were too poor to afford housing when they needed it. The largest number (27%) reported abuse as the event triggering their need, followed by eviction (22%), separation (14%), pregnancy (11%), and overcrowding (9%). Once housing became affordable through housing subsidies, these former guests showed they were able to keep it: 94% remained housed after leaving Wellspring (Quiñones, 1992).

## Attitudes Toward Poverty

These are the facts about the poverty and homelessness of American mothers and their children (and it should be noted that in 1995 one American child in five lived in poverty; no other industrialized nation comes even close to this shameful figure; Bassuk et al., 1996). But Americans' ideas about poverty remain singularly resistant to facts. Repeated polls and surveys have shown that we, unlike citizens of other industrialized nations, blame poverty on the poor themselves: "In keeping with the dominant American belief system," says Wilson (1996), "it is the moral fabric of individuals, not the social and economic structure of society, that is taken to be the root of the problem."

> "I sit there and criticize myself. . . . I messed up, I screwed up, this is my fault. If I had tried a little harder, maybe if I had got two jobs instead of one job."

As women who have worked with homeless mothers for more than 25 years among us, we reject this view of the roots of mothers' homelessness. We believe that social, political, and economic factors far beyond individuals' control create poverty, and we believe poverty creates the homelessness of mothers. We saw the increase in homelessness that paralleled the drastic federal reduction of commitment to low-cost housing beginning in the 1980s; we expect to see far worse under the full impact of recent changes in welfare programs.

Bassuk et al.'s (1996) Worcester research supports this view. Despite finding "shocking" levels of physical and sexual assault and their emotional aftermath among homeless mothers (91.6% reported past physical or sexual assaults; Bassuk et al., 1996), researchers stated categorically that economic factors—not the mothers' mental health difficulties, their compromised physical health, violence and its aftermath, "welfare dependency," or the "culture of poverty"—but economic factors were responsible for mothers becoming homeless (Bassuk et al., 1996).

This research is a welcome confirmation of our experience. We do not deny the importance of individuals' choices and actions in determining some of the circumstances of their lives. But we see that terrible events strike not only homeless mothers we have worked with, but also economically better-off women, even the wealthy and famous. We see the bad decisions made by politicians our society lionizes, by celebrities it idealizes, by sports figures it canonizes—and by homeless mothers it demonizes. The difference we see is that those who became homeless lacked financial and personal resources to protect themselves and their children from the worst consequences of their actions. Their difficulties become public property, subject to public censure, because they are dependent on public support. Those who have the resources to hide their misfortunes do not risk such social opprobrium.

Clearly, we reject the idea that homeless mothers are inherently "dysfunctional" women, requiring an array of services and supports so they can become "good" mothers. Rather, we believe they are women who have faced violence—perhaps physical violence, perhaps the violence only of poverty—without the protection of adequate resources. For some, the simple act of gaining access to affordable housing is enough to allow them to return to lives that conform to our society's picture of adequate motherhood. But many others enter shelter in a state of deep disorganization. They may be in shock over the violence they have suffered. They may be profoundly grieving the loss of home, family, friends, neighborhood. They may have faced lifelong poverty and abuse or only recent incidents of it; they may have faced a cascade of unanticipated events or a sudden disaster. Whatever their circumstances, as they enter shelter they have very often been robbed not only of their homes but also of precisely the abilities most needed to cope with the social condemnation and lack of resources they now face.

## LOSING HOME, FINDING HOME

"Because I'm homeless, that don't make me a bad mother."

For many mothers, homelessness is a reality long before they join the statistics of families who are "officially" homeless—those who have received formal public assistance to pay for emergency housing in a shelter or motel. Before taking this step, many mothers and their families live for a time with parents, other relatives, or friends. As one Wellspring guest described it, a mother avoiding entering emergency shelter will "bounce your kid from here to there. . . . I'll stay there for a couple of weeks . . . that don't work out, and so you end up somewhere else, and that don't work out and you're somewhere else. . . . " Although not "officially" homeless while this is going on, can this mother truly be said to have a home? Or, if in a shelter a mother is able to establish what Ruddick (1989) calls a home—a "headquarters for a mother's organizing and a child's growing"—then what does it mean to be "officially" homeless? For that matter, in this context what is a mother's "home"? Does it require a house or apartment? Or is it any place where she can perform the tasks central to mothering—the preservation of her children's safety, the nurturing of their growth, and the fostering of their social acceptability (Ruddick, 1989)? We must, it seems, look beyond the traditional notion of "home" to understand our own setting.

Wellspring's seven founders chose to make a home together to share with people in need. They understood living together in community to be essential for practicing their radical vision of hospitality. After 16 years, two of Wellspring's founders still make their home in this old house and continue to share it with homeless families. In other words, the same home contains some people who are "housed" and others who are "homeless." For none of them is this "home" in the traditional sense. Meals are prepared by staff and volunteers and taken in common at fixed times; volunteers and staff take on most household duties in common areas. The corporation, not those who live in it, owns the home. The homeless families sheltered there, originally called "community members," chose instead to call themselves "guests" to acknowledge differences in status and power between themselves and those who reside there of their own positive choice. Founders and staff accepted the term, with its connotations of guests as honored, if transient, residents who bring gifts as well as receive hospitality.

Our guests are engaged in precisely those mothering tasks that would normally go on within the confines of a "home." This home, however, is a temporary one by its very definition as a "family shelter." Shelter staff must attempt to help guests understand that they can carry many aspects of "home" with them when they leave the shelter, that, in an image used by Lewis, they can be like mother hens, fluffing up their feathers wherever they may be, to provide safety and warmth to their chicks. Home, Lewis tells them, can be truly "under our feathers." For us, the challenge is to help them create a "home" that will survive the experiences of both being in and moving out of shelter.

## Examining Mothering and Homelessness

We began our work on this chapter by convening two focus groups, one of guests then in our shelter and one of former guests. The voices scattered through this chapter come from both. The identified conversations all originated with the mothers in the latter group, women at some remove from their homeless experience. Names and identifying details have been altered to disguise these mothers' identities.

- Josie grew up in a working-class, two-parent home with an alcoholic father. Her marriage to a "professional" seemed ideal until his sexual demands began to include putting on diapers and playing at being a child; he locked her in a closet for hours when she refused to participate. Eventually, Josie and the two children fled to her parents' home, and Josie filed for divorce. When tensions became unbearable with her mother, Josie and her children came to Wellspring. Almost immediately, the children disclosed being sexually abused by their father. The family subsequently went through countless hours of counseling and court involvement. Returning from court-ordered visitation, the children continued to relay to Josie their father's death threats. Throughout this period and through the time of this writing, Josie has maintained an excellent work record.

- Sara and her brother were abandoned by their mother as young children; her addict father was unaware of Sara's sexual abuse by her brother. Her early marriage to a nonsmoking teetotaler was an attempt to create safe boundaries, but 5 years later he had become drug dependent and violent. Sara and her two children arrived at the shelter after her daycare provider quit without notice, depriving her of her job and the salary to pay for an apartment. Now in a stable second marriage, Sara is currently on staff at a social service agency.

- Claire grew up in a family dominated by her father's violence and addictions. Claire herself was hospitalized for depression and anxiety following the discovery that her children's father was having an affair. He subsequently refused to allow her to return to the home she had paid for. She and her two children came into shelter after several cramped months with relatives.

- Christine's large, apparently normal middle-class family was in reality a tangle of sexual and emotional abuse. Until her teens, Christine believed that her mother was her sister and that her grandmother was her mother, learning the truth only on her grandmother's death. At 19, Christine also learned that her mother/sister was having an affair with the father of Christine's unborn child. Left without the support of boyfriend or family, Christine went into shelter with her newborn. Ten years later, Christine still finds it hard at times to "stay in my body." She no longer drives because of at least two accidents while in this trauma-related dissociated state.

"Sometimes my mother would come over. Every once in a while she'd come over to bring a gift or something. She'd say, 'You should put your kids in foster homes. . . . You don't have nothing to give them, you're stressed out, you can't do it.' "

We cannot say these women are "typical." We have worked with professional ballerinas, college graduates, women who never completed the sixth grade. Although they are overwhelmingly white, our guests have also been African American and Hispanic; immigrants and old New England stock; impressively eloquent in English and speakers only of other languages. Many stories are much worse than these we have told; a few are better. But we do not find the experiences of these four women to be unusual.

Nevertheless, as we listen to their stories we are repeatedly awestruck. We ask ourselves whether, denied necessary resources, we could preserve a family while being simultaneously bombarded with messages of blame, of incompetence, of society's belief that we cannot—indeed, should not—do so. Yet our guests do survive their homelessness with dignity and strength, they maintain their family life, and some thrive once they have established a new home. And so we asked: How do they manage this? Where do they find the strengths to struggle against both external and internal judgments about their situations, their decisions, their selves?

## THE ROLE OF RESISTANCE

Fundamental to this ability is the cultivation and nurturing of resistance. By this we mean the ability to resist the messages that bombard them, both internally and externally, that they are not doing their jobs as mothers, that they are neither good mothers nor even good-enough mothers, that they deserve to feel as they do: degraded, ashamed, failed. "When I was in the shelter, when I was scrambling to try to make the next meal on the table and stuff, I felt lost and useless and degraded and like there was nothing out there for me," Sara recalled. Yet she and each one of the other guests and former guests we spoke to located the source of their resistance to these feelings in precisely the same place others find much of their shame: being mothers.

"Your kids keep you going," Josie declared.

"'Cause your kids are all you have," agreed Christine. "The fact that you're so important to them keeps you going. . . . Sometimes it gets to the point you think if you give them up they'd be better off. But you don't, 'cause then you'd have no control over what happens to them. There's a lot sicker things that could happen besides being poor and not having anything."

In other words, it is precisely their experience as mothers that these women use as their compass, orienting them as they resist negative messages, or as they internalize the messages and resist them nonetheless. As mothers, they see the vilified option of "official" homelessness as preferable to either surviving continued violence or navigating from friend to relative, relative to friend. As mothers, they confront and struggle through the pain not only of their current, socially condemned situation but also of their own pasts, in order to provide a home for their families.

> "Regardless of what everybody else thinks, you know that you're taking care of your child the proper way. . . . It just kicks in, you know, that the child comes first, and if you want to be a good mother, you've got to make right decisions."

In formulating our thoughts about resistance, we found especially useful Robinson and Ward's (1991) discussion, developed in the context of African American adolescents. They identify two stages: resistance for survival, or the short-term and sometimes self-destructive strategies that permit survival in a hostile and oppressive environment; and resistance for liberation, the act of confronting the realities of and demanding change in that environment.

We are working with women who have similar but not identical issues. Wellspring guests are with a few exceptions white, they are older than adolescent, they are mothers. Their ethnic identities seldom permit their connection to traditional African philosophies that Robinson and Ward (1991) use to construct a new model of resistance. Furthermore, their patterns of resistance are frequently complicated by trauma, an issue that will be covered more thoroughly later in this chapter. Therefore, although we are indebted to Robinson and Ward's (1991) framework, we use a slightly different rubric comprising three forms of resistance: resistance for survival, resistance for equality, and resistance for transformation.

We borrow the term "transformation" from the late Brazilian educator Paulo Freire (1993), who argued that only the oppressed (and those in solidarity with them) can change the nature of their relationship with their oppressors. In order to make change, the oppressed "must perceive the reality of oppression not as a closed world from which there is no exit, but as a limiting situation which they can transform" (Freire, 1993, p. 31). Transformation, as distinct from liberation, involves casting out the oppressor within as well as challenging the oppressor without. When we are doing our best work, we are helping mothers achieve "critical consciousness" (in Freire's words) of both oppressive external forces and limiting and destructive internal states. The next challenge is to help them with strategies for actual changes. (For more discussion of these points, see the introduction to this book.)

In the sections that follow, we describe resistance for survival, resistance for equality, and resistance for transformation as three separate stages, but they are not discrete phases in a neat progression. The mothers we work with often use strategies of one, two, or three forms of resistance simultaneously, or they may oscillate back and forth among them.

## Resistance for Survival and Resistance for Equality

When mothers first leave their homes, their overriding aim is survival for themselves and their children. Bouncing from place to place, doubling up with parents or relatives, or other forms of temporary shelter can be seen as resistance for survival: resistance to the demeaning label of "homeless" with all its connotations about their abilities as mothers. As the women in our focus groups so poignantly reminded us, at this point their identity as mothers is very nearly their only possession. Threats to it are not taken lightly. But this and other strategies "undertaken solely to maintain survival can represent dysfunctional adaptations to an oppressive reality and tend only to provide short term relief" (Robinson & Ward, 1991, p. 90). For homeless mothers, being transient ultimately proves costly to the very identity so important to them.

> "I did everything I could to stay out of a shelter, but it happened. It was either that or keep bringing my kid to this one's house and that one's house, and that's not good for the child. I think that my real mothering skills kicked in. It's like, she needs stableness, and I need to give it to her now."

We see the act of entering shelter as an act of resistance for both survival and equality. A mother places herself and her children at the mercy of a system she may desperately fear, and that by its very nature degrades her. But in doing so, she also makes a claim—conscious or not—that she feels herself and her children to be as deserving of available community resources as others have been. It is this claim that we call resistance for equality.

But the costs to this step are almost inconceivably painful and may well be part of the way in which becoming homeless produces its own trauma. First is the knowledge that by entering a shelter system that may place her literally anywhere in the state, she will certainly face the loss of whatever home she has been able to provide, and possibly as well the loss of a familiar and perhaps beloved neighborhood, the loss of friends, of family, of her own autonomy. And there is always the terrible fear that no matter what decision she makes, she may lose her children. Recalled one guest of her decision to seek shelter, "I thought they were going to take my kid away from me. I really believed that they were going to snatch my child away." Another immediately responded with fear grounded in the only alternative action: "I figured if I keep bouncing my kids from house to house without a stable place to live, they was going to take my kids."

But there is still more cost to come. To qualify for emergency shelter, a mother must prove to a welfare worker that she literally has nowhere else to go. She must list friends and relatives and show, often in writing, that each has refused her shelter. The worker may telephone those listed to request shelter for the family. If anyone grants it, whether on beds, couches, or a floor, *and even if only for that one night,* the application is denied. Thus the process for entering emergency shelter forces a mother to choose between the transient life she knows is damaging to her children, and the graphic demonstration that all of her relationships, connections, supports—partner, parents, family, friends—have rejected her.

"It's like you're giving up everything. You're giving up everything."

Nevertheless, we believe that the decision to enter shelter may represent positive movement, a mother's decision to look further ahead than this one night. Once in the shelter, mothers continue establishing safety and legal equality with restraining orders, custody arrangements, and visitation; advocating for themselves and their children with various government bodies (courts, schools, welfare agencies, housing authorities); and getting improved health and mental health care.

Taking these steps of resistance for equality, however, does not mean shelter guests shed all manifestations of resistance for survival. We often see guests' survival strategies surface in hostility to the requirements of congregate living: to rules, to group meetings, and to maintaining their own and others' privacy, calm, and quiet. Survival strategies may also present as emotional numbing, denial, anger, isolation, or, on the more positive side, maintaining connections with family and friends even though they may be judgmental and unsupportive.

> "I get a lot of criticism, especially from family members. They say, 'You're so strong, you've always taken care of yourself, why are you in a shelter now?' "

Continuation of resistance for survival may be particularly evident in defensive responses to staff advice or suggestions on parenting issues, which unless carefully presented can be understood as additional messages that they are not good mothers. All of this, we believe, represents not the reactivity of a "dysfunctional" individual, but rather a mother's attempt to resist the unrelenting challenges to her own identity as a mother.

## Trauma

For many, these issues revolve around past trauma. We must here make the distinction between the effects of marginalization and those of trauma. The women we work with are all marginalized—they lack necessary resources to conform to a societal ideal of the "good mother." They have been rendered powerless and voiceless. They are at the mercy of systems they can neither understand nor control; they hear all around them other voices speaking ugly and unrecognizable descriptions of themselves and their reality. Their efforts at resisting injury from this assault are evident in alienation, fear, isolation, refusal to connect with others, or inability to take advantage of the community resources available. Unmasking this marginalization and helping them find more effective means to combat it are difficult enough.

But from evidence already presented, it is clear that a large majority of women and children entering shelter have experienced severe trauma in their lives. Thus they may demonstrate a heightened level of psychological injury. Some symptoms of trauma may not differ in nature from those of marginalization, but they will certainly differ in their higher degree of intensity. The guests may also have additional cognitive and neurological complications. For some, the experience of homelessness itself may be the primary trauma. Living in shelter, Goodman, Saxe, and Harvey (1991, p. 1219) suggest, "with such attendant stressors as the possible loss of safety, predictability and control—may undermine and finally erode coping capabilities and precipitate symptoms of psychological trauma" for both individuals and families. For others who have previously been able to banish them, symptoms from prior traumatic incidents may be aggravated or reactivated by the stress of their homelessness (Goodman et al., 1991).

In either case, symptoms of trauma may include flashbacks and dissociation; emotional numbing and increased arousal (irritability, angry outbursts, hypervigilance, sleep disturbances); substance abuse; self-mutilation; intolerance of intimacy; a sense of helplessness, isolation, and separateness. Significantly for our work, it also can induce feelings of social disaffiliation, of "being without sanctuary in a world filled with malevolent forces" (Goodman et al., 1991, p. 1220). These trauma issues and the process of recovery from them, interwoven with whatever positive adaptations a mother is trying to make, complicate enormously the already daunting tasks confronting both the mother who finds herself homeless and those who work with her. For those who are able to begin it, however, recovery from trauma involves three stages of healing, according to Judith Herman (1992): first of creating a sense of safety and control, then a period of remembrance and mourning, and finally the move toward establishing reconnection.

In the Wellspring shelter, the first necessity for all new guests is the creation of physical safety. The front door is always locked; staff and volunteers screen phone calls and refuse them from abusers. Rules and routines—eating, sleeping, laundry, quiet times—help guests recover a sense of control over their lives. But chaos may have had a survival function of fending off emotional pain, and thus guests do not always relinquish the chaos without a struggle. Guests often resist shelter rules, complain that they are too strict, violate them in secret, pit one worker's interpretation of the rules against another's, jeopardize their own and their children's safety by contacting abusers and sometimes even sneaking out to see them. We can now see these familiar actions as strategies of resistance for survival. That this resistance becomes no less exasperating and exhausting for staff through this understanding is a fact of shelter work.

But congregate living of necessity requires guidelines. And as the mothers' understanding of rules begins to reduce the chaos that formerly kept at bay the memory or, in some cases, the acknowledgment of trauma, the hidden feelings that have so shaped their lives may begin to rise into consciousness. Confronting past trauma can itself feel like a threat to survival, and so these mothers may face yet another terrible dilemma: Is it better to mother minimally, using much of their energy to maintain the chaos that keeps emotion away, or to drown in the flood they fear will be unleashed by facing the trauma, and not be able to mother at all?

> "I remember saying to somebody when I was leaving the shelter, that all the things they try to teach you when you're there are very important, valid things, assertiveness and stuff like that. But I feel like at a time in your life when everything is so haywire and you don't even know what you're doing the next minute, it's really hard to try to learn all these new behaviorisms, these new things, when you're just trying to function, [in] day-to-day life."

But it is during this time of simultaneously establishing and resisting safety, control, and order that the second stage of trauma recovery—remembrance and mourning—often begins. Guests may begin to feel among themselves and staff the construction of a network of supports and relationships to replace the one so dramatically demolished in the process of becoming homeless. Within the safety of that network, the stability of that routine, recovery may proceed.

> "As I went into the shelter, I found out that with my marriage, I had been very traumatized . . . it all came out at the shelter. I never thought being in the shelter was going to lead to what it led to. Finding things out that you ignore, and you hide, and—'No, no, it can't be, no, shut up,' you know what I mean? . . . And then you find out that the person you were married to . . . did something to your kids. . . . The shelter was positive as far as getting the support and the help and the awareness of what is actually going on in your life, that I kept shutting out. 'No, I won't think about that.' . . . I didn't want to let it in."

Josie, who related this story during our focus group with former guests, did finally "let it in." Her courageous act of maternal protection and the consequences that followed it demonstrate the costs homeless mothers may face as they break through one level of resistance to another: the possibility that they will have to confront the terrible truths of their lives.

## Resistance for Transformation

While guests are in our shelter, much of our work necessarily revolves around issues of survival and equality. Much of this is empowering. We see guests growing in confidence and power by taking control of their housing search and budgeting, of personal and relational growth in shelter group meetings, of learning to be supported in a community while they advocate for themselves with other agencies or appeal adverse decisions from them. When we have done our best work, guests may reach a critical moment when they begin to understand that Wellspring is committed to being partners in resistance rather than a party to their oppression. This work helps guests identify the tools for creating both a new way of being in the world and a new world to be in—in short, a vision of transformation.

Transformation, however—the ability to think and act in ways that change reality for oneself and for one's society—is not a quick process. During shelter stays that average 6 months (as of early 1998), the seeds we plant will not bear their fruit, either for the mothers themselves or for the society around them. And so we face a dilemma: While mothers are in shelter, we must offer them the tools to begin moving toward transformation. However, in the midst of overwhelming tasks of survival and equality—as well as a cycle of housing availability unrelated to the timing of their personal tasks—we must not expect guests to master these tools. To do so is to court predictable disappointment, to risk a return to blaming mothers for not achieving unachievable goals.

When guests do move in the direction of transformation, however, the result can be a powerful shift in consciousness. Guests who participate in political actions aimed at changing the society that oppresses them—lobbying at the State House, giving interviews to the media, speaking out in other public forums—are claiming and pro-claiming the value of their lives and experience. They tell us that these are among the most empowering events of their time with us. But for some mothers, it may take years after leaving the shelter before they can begin to name stereotypes and actively refuse them, to reject or force change in relationships that reinforce stereotypes in favor of others fostering growth. We watch, and aid them as we can, as they acquire, use, and create education to promote justice for women, as they develop or join existing community programs aimed at economic and/or social justice, speak out publicly, lobby for improved legislation.

And we observe as well the costs and consequences of their acts of transformation. Family ties and old friendships may be broken, finding new relationships with either other women or men may be difficult, and daring to speak out publicly may bring swift reprisal.

> "I was in one of [author] Wendy's groups . . . and all the welfare reform changes were going on. You wanted us to write to the president. . . . I did, and I got a letter back. . . . He said in his letter, 'We want people to understand that they should not have children until they're prepared to take care of them.' That was in the letter from the president."

Neither Christine, who told this story in our focus group, nor the rest of us listening were willing to accept this simplistic vision of an always predictable life. Christine herself had only just finished saying how clearly that same message had reached her when she was homeless, when family and friends were urging her to give up her children. Being homeless meant that "you don't have the right to have kids that you can't take care of," she had said. "You did wrong even to have the kids, because you don't have the means to support them. Regardless of the situation when you had the kid, you should have been able to foresee the future, that there was a point that you wouldn't be able to take care of them."

These were no longer simply words to be examined for objective meaning. The setting had opened us, and we all, authors included, could imagine ourselves in Christine's position, homeless and abandoned, experiencing our own emotions upon being told that we should never have had our own children. These words from the President of the United States stunned us, becoming a powerful blow to an already shaky hold on being an adequate mother. We all leaped to support Christine. "I would have just mailed it back to him," declared Sara, "saying, 'Where's your crystal ball?' " She laughed as she spoke, and we began to join her. This intense moment of shared outrage and laughter knit us together. As mothers together, we could name and resist the culturally sanctioned myth. We could share belief in the truth we knew. For that moment we could be sustained by a vision of even the distant possibility of transformation, powerfully shared.

But amidst the daily demands of survival and equality, how do we sustain that vision?

## COMMUNITIES OF RESISTANCE

The answer, we believe, lies precisely in the interaction just described: the creation of what Welch (1985) calls "communities of resistance."

Such a community helps us to name and define the forces that marginalize us; it voices a definition of its members that affirms, supports, and includes us all in the whole body of human experience. And as the term "communities of resistance" so aptly suggests, resistance—whether to misfortune, marginalization, or oppression—is most likely to be successful when undertaken in community. Standing alone, no one of us has the resources to resist a hurricane; together, we can create mutual shelter.

For us as workers, the Wellspring organization has provided that community of resistance. We stand outside our society's mainstream of beliefs about poverty and homelessness, and about the appropriate ways of working with mothers who have become homeless. Believing profoundly in the need for systemic social change, we often find ourselves, our beliefs, and our practices minimized and marginalized. Maintaining our beliefs and our ability to practice them has required just such a sheltering community.

## IMPLICATIONS FOR PRACTICE

In the process of working with the ideas in this chapter, we, the authors, have felt ourselves and our understanding of our work to be deeply changed. We are able now to understand familiar dynamics in a new way, and we have begun to identify areas most likely to be influenced by the examination we have undertaken.

1. First, we must hold mothering at the center of our framework. When we describe actions and attitudes as "mothering," we are not saying that they are performed only by women, or only by women who have borne children. We mean rather that mothering as a practice, especially its nurturing, growth-fostering core, has traditionally been conceptualized as a female attribute. We believe with Ruddick that "a mother is a person who takes on responsibility for children's lives and for whom providing child care is a significant part of her or his working life" (Ruddick, 1989, p. 40). All shelter staff—male, female, mothers, nonmothers, grandmothers—have mothering tasks as part of their work. But for the single parents we work with, their tasks of mothering are the core of their lives.

"What kept me going was the happy times. . . . I felt like everyone had left me, but I still had my baby, and it was cozy, and he was healthy, and he was adorable, and I could still do that right."

At the least, shelter staff must never lose sight of this mothering core; at the most, we must join guests there for true empathy. We must find more ways to use this perspective in the way that homeless mothers do. When we use our own mothering practice as a candle to illuminate the shadowy corners of our work and relationships with them, we experience an extraordinary shift in both perception and position. In our focus groups, inhabiting our own core identities as mothers opened a powerful experience of mutuality among all of us present. In Judith Jordan's words, we were "both affecting each other and being affected by each other," we were open to "influence, emotional availability, and a constantly changing pattern of responding to and affecting [each] other's state" (Jordan, 1991, p. 82). No longer "expert" and "client," "knowing staff" and "unknowing guest," we experienced a diminution of the identities (privilege, education, race, authority) that normally divide us and that set up the familiar oppressive dynamic of power and resistance. We were all called to experience an unfamiliar state, to leave comfortable roles behind—even if only for a moment—and enter an intense shared connection that simultaneously challenged and sustained us as we changed, learned, and grew. Understanding and acknowledging this dynamic and consciously establishing mutuality can be a powerful tool for our work.

For example, in attempting to resolve repeated petty rules violations with one guest, Lewis found that when she imagined and allowed herself to experience her own feelings as a mother in the guest's circumstances, it became quite clear that the rules violations were a symbol of a larger problem. This mother might be unable to ward off other blows—the homelessness itself, the ongoing resistance of the larger system to providing what she and her family needed—but resisting shelter rules was one available way to fight for her survival as a mother. From within this experience, Lewis and the guest could move into solidarity as mothers, and begin to examine ways of moving out of resistance for survival and into resistance for equality—perhaps even for transformation.

2. We have seen the critical importance of developing communities of resistance. We see guests and former guests forming communities of resistance to help them overcome the obstacles confronting them as they move toward transformation. The focus groups we convened appeared to function in that manner, with participants both joining in community in the moment and reflecting on other, similar experiences. Focusing on motherhood allowed us to move beyond the role of simple support and into resistance. Together, we could all confront the stark

contradiction between society's description of homeless mothers and our own lived experience. Together, we were able to name and clarify negative messages, the better to resist them.

> "I've always believed I was a rock. You just can't throw me on the ground and crack me right away. . . . But I always needed someone there to remind me. . . . I needed somebody to remind me of that all the time."

We have also seen the consequences for workers of the lack of such communities. In our experience of shelters and agencies, those most likely to be working in the most difficult situations with homeless mothers are often the least trained, least experienced, and least rewarded (financially and otherwise) of all their colleagues. The results of this are plain in interactions with those they attempt to serve. An example was one extremely difficult conference with a guest who was being required to leave our shelter for hospitalization. Lewis could remain in close, caring relationship, believing in the guest's essential value as person and as mother while telling her she must leave, because Lewis is surrounded by supportive coworkers. Also present was a worker from a large state agency. This worker, alone in coping with the emotionally brutal task of moving a child into foster care, visibly withdrew from any relationship, refusing to answer questions and recoiling in disgust when Lewis hugged the mother. Here, truly, is resistance for survival: the worker's resistance to being drawn into another's pain for the sake of her own survival. We discover this resistance in ourselves as well when we are overtaxed and isolated, when we too give in to the judgments that allow us to keep a safe distance from the pain of the women we work with. But we believe that this refusal of mutual relationship is deeply destructive to our work. Our own community of resistance helps us resist pressures for distance so we can, in Lewis's words, walk with other mothers through "the dark and scary places" we all encounter on the path to transformation.

3. This path toward transformation is often a difficult one to find, and an even more difficult one to support with resources and funds. If we want guests to go to meetings with legislators, for example, staff must arrange childcare, coordinate schedules for children's school and mothers' travel, cancel or reschedule required shelter activities. We must often overcome guests' understandable reluctance to confront powerful people in unfamiliar settings. We must make the time to work with guests for many hours, helping them prepare and rehearse

questions that they will feel confident enough to ask, stories they will feel strong enough to tell. And we must do this knowing that children's illnesses, sudden demands for meetings with other agencies, unexpected housing opportunities, or other last-minute emergencies can mean all of our effort goes for naught. Nevertheless, if we believe that these are activities that truly move guests toward transformation, we must find ways to support them more effectively.

4. We must accept the idea that in a relational context, both parties must move toward transformation. For staff, this means training in social analysis, in sharing the understanding of their own experience in a historical and cultural context. In an organizational sense, this means building structures that include in decisions both guests and participants in Wellspring's other programs—sharing power, in short. We must intentionally include former guests and program participants on boards or management teams, if necessary changing meeting dynamics or offering training so they can play active rather than token roles. Achieving this transformative process requires staff to view themselves as "animators," helping guests "to 'unveil' their situation" (Hope & Timmel, 1984, p. 14), to examine and analyze the contradictions between their everyday experience and the dictates of the dominant cultural paradigm, and to take action based on this new understanding.

5. Last, and most fundamental to our practice, both guests and former guests clearly voiced what they must have from us who work with them, if they are to undertake what Freire (1993, p. 26) calls "the vocation of becoming more fully human": to ask rather than assume, to listen rather than direct, to respect rather than judge.

> "I want to be treated like I treat others. And I'm always treating everybody with respect. Even the worst of people. My mother always said, 'Kill them with kindness, period.' When I don't get that respect I start to get really disappointed and I become depressed. . . . I mean, I feel degraded."

When Sara skips a required shelter meeting to take her children to the park, we can stop for a moment before we accuse her of "oppositional" behavior and ask her why she missed the meeting. We would then learn that after many hours with her small children in district court obtaining a restraining order, this mother felt her family would benefit more from some happy time together than from separating the children to daycare while she attended a meeting. When

Claire invites an alcoholic man to move in with her for a time, we can stop for a moment before we label her behavior "immoral" and ask her why she has done this. We would then learn that this mother sought protection from a former husband who continued to believe he had rights not only to his children but also to her. As soon as the ex gets the (false) message that she is someone else's property, the alcoholic guest is gone. When Christine, whose trauma from childhood sexual abuse often brings on dissociative states, speaks of frequent marijuana smoking, we can stop for a moment before we condemn her "antisocial" or "pathological" behavior and ask her why she does it. We would then learn that marijuana helps this mother stay present to her children.

These clearly are not ideal strategies for reaching the goals these mothers aim for, nor are they strategies that we initially recognized as reflective of strength and courage rather than of weakness and dysfunction. We hope that now we can help these mothers find ways of reaching their goals in ways that produce fewer negative side effects. If we *ask* why mothers have undertaken these behaviors, if we *listen* while they tell us, if we *respect* their goals, perhaps we can walk the path toward transformation together.

These points are deceptively simple. But the pressures of day-to-day practice and sheer magnitude of need among the women we work with challenge our ability to hold firmly to this new framework. Nevertheless, we find that the more we are able to maintain our commitment to the centrality of mothering, the more we discover new strategies for meeting not only homeless mothers' goals of caring well for their families, but our own of moving toward a fairer and more just society as well.

## REFERENCES

Bassuk, E. L., Browne, A., & Buckner, J. C. (1996). Single mothers and welfare. *Scientific American, 275*(4), 60–67.

Freire, P. (1993). *Pedagogy of the oppressed* (rev. ed.). New York: Continuum.

Goodman, L., Saxe, L., & Harvey, M. (1991). Homelessness as psychological trauma. *American Psychologist 46*(11), 1219–1225.

Herman, J. L. (1992). *Trauma and recovery.* New York: Basic Books.

Hope, A., & Timmel, S. (1984). *Training for transformation: A handbook for community workers. Book I.* Gweru, Zimbabwe: Mambo Press.

Jordan, J. V. (1991). The meaning of mutuality. In J. V. Jordan, A. G. Kaplan,

J. B. Miller, I. P. Stiver, & J. L. Surrey, *Women's growth in connection: Writings from the Stone Center* (pp. 81–96). New York: Guilford Press.

National Coalition for the Homeless. (1996). *Why are people homeless?* Washington, DC: Author.

Quiñones, W. (1992). Let them have housing. *New England Journal of Public Policy, 8*(1), 557–581.

Robinson, T., & Ward, V. W. (1991). "A belief in self far greater than anyone's disbelief": Cultivating resistance among African American female adolescents. In C. Gilligan, A. G. Rogers, & D. L. Tolman (Eds.), *Women, girls, and psychotherapy: Reframing resistance* (pp. 87–104). Binghamton, NY: Harrington Park Press.

Ruddick, S. (1989). *Maternal thinking: Toward a politics of peace.* Boston: Beacon Press.

U.S. Conference of Mayors. (1996). *A status report on hunger and homelessness in America's Cities: 1996.* Washington, DC: Author.

Welch, S. (1985). *Communities of resistance and solidarity: A feminist theology of liberation.* New York: Orbis Books.

Wilson, W. J. (1996). *When work disappears: The world of the new urban poor.* New York: Knopf.

# 4

## Immigrant Mothers
### What Makes Them High Risk?

*MARILYN G. FRAKTMAN*

*THE* act of leaving one's country is neither simple nor easy. It can be wrought with emotions of loss, grief, anxiety, high expectations, and hope. When immigration is followed by the birth of a baby, especially to first-time parents, a new burden of conflicting emotions can be added. This latter burden is not unique to immigrants. The parents' joy and exhilaration are joined by high levels of stress, heightened anxiety, and disequilibrium. These stresses include physiological stress (Blackburn, 1992; Rose & Ginnetty, 1989) and psychosocial stress (Gladieux, 1978; Belsky & Rovine, 1984; Belsky & Kelly, 1994). New parents often refer to being caught off balance, which requires some degree of adaptation (Plutzik & Laghi, 1983). In extreme cases, especially in the early postpartum phase, clinical depression may be diagnosed (Mammen, 1993; Stern & Kruckman, 1983).

In spite of parents' conflicting emotions, the early postpartum period has been identified as an important time for growth and development (Weingarten & Daniels, 1983). However, resources that can enhance parent learning and provide emotional support are often unavailable or inaccessible. Many parents receive little or no information during the postpartum period to assist them in the psychological, physical, or emotional transitions that accompany bringing home a new baby (Ewy & Youmans, 1988). The provision of meaningful support services in the immediate postpartum phase to ameliorate some of these stresses has continued to focus primarily on "high-risk" populations. Immigrant mothers, usually of color, with English as their second language, are frequently grouped into this category. The "high-risk" label carries an implicit criticism of immigrant mothers at the same time that it makes them eligible for support services immediately after birth, services that are not widely available to U.S.-born mothers.

## KNOWLEDGE DEFICIT: INFANT AT RISK

As a visiting nurse I have repeatedly seen the diagnosis *knowledge deficit* on referrals. This diagnosis is often assigned to immigrant mothers. What knowledge the mother is specifically deficient in is not clearly defined. In some instances, a poor command of the English language supports the assumption of deficiency. What usually accompanies this diagnosis is either a secondary diagnosis or an assumption: infant at risk. The risk to the infant is also not explicit. Inferred in that diagnosis is the idea that the baby is at risk for either a compromised health outcome or abuse and neglect, which is implied to stem from the mother's "knowledge" deficiency.

But, just how "deficient" are immigrant first-time mothers compared to their U.S.-born counterparts? I would like to illustrate two separate referrals sent to two different agencies.

### Referral 1

Sally, a native born U.S. citizen, was a first-time mother, approximately 35 years of age, married for about 5 years, and previously a professional. She had delivered her first baby by cesarean. She planned to breastfeed her baby. She had had no previous experience with breastfeeding or caring for infants and, in particular, newborns. She and her husband lived in their own home in a suburb west of Boston. She was discharged from the hospital after a 3-day stay. The referral from the insurance company requested a postpartum evaluation for the mother and newborn. The purpose of the nursing visit was to assess both Sally's and her baby's physical status. In addition, Sally's health insurance benefit qualified her to receive a highly restrictive, time-limited home health service.

### Referral 2

Claudia was a first-time mother, approximately 35 years old, married for about 5 years, and living with her husband in an apartment in a small city outside of Boston. She was not a professional; instead, she immigrated to the United States approximately 5 years earlier. Claudia spoke a limited amount of English. She had delivered her first baby by cesarean and planned to breastfeed her infant. She had had no prior experience with breastfeeding or caring for infants and, in particular, newborns. She was discharged from the hospital after a 3-day stay. The referral was made by Claudia's physician who requested a postpartum evaluation of her and her baby. The diagnosis on this referral read: knowledge deficit. The number and frequency of scheduled home visits were to be determined from the evaluation and in collaboration with the patient.

When one compares these two referrals one sees more similarities than differences. However, Claudia, who is an immigrant as well as a new mother, has been labeled. She will be more carefully followed and possibly scrutinized for her parenting ability because of her immigrant status, which is accentuated by her limited ability to speak English. Is Sally more capable? It appears that she possesses the same knowledge deficit for parenting and breastfeeding her newborn as Claudia. In fact, research (Fraktman, 1997) indicates that all first-time parents experience knowledge deficit in parenting and breastfeeding their newborns. In my recently completed study, all of the 15 participating couples, who were first-time parents, admitted that they lacked knowledge in newborn care and breastfeeding. These participants constituted a mature, one might say privileged, group, with an educational range from high school diploma to master's degree.

Although a referral activates a supportive intervention, the diagnosis of *knowledge deficit,* by definition, creates an image of deficiency, with the potential to cause harm to both mother and child. The practice of labeling people rather than assessing their needs marginalizes their experience by placing a deficit framework on inexperience and so actively encourages discriminatory practices. Providers thus may look for differences and deficits rather than strengths and competencies. The diagnosis also is entered into medical records and influences all future treatment.

If the purpose of the referral is to support immigrant women who are without family members in this country, to teach and assist them in caring for their newborn and help them access services, one would expect that most, if not all, immigrant women, especially those who are first-time mothers, would qualify for such services. This, however, does not seem to be the case. As a nurse, I visit many immigrant women following their discharge after the delivery of their baby. I

would like to share the story of two immigrant women who participated in my research. One woman had been in this country less than
1 year and the other for 5 years. Both were first-time mothers. They
openly discussed the fact that they had no experience caring for infants
and no knowledge of breastfeeding. They did not have any extended
family in the country to provide postpartum support. Both women
were white. One was a native English speaker. The other woman, for
whom English was her second language, spoke with a heavy accent.
One woman had received some formal education beyond high school.
The other woman had a master's degree in nursing.

One was not referred for any postpartum services. The other
received one home visit, which was part of a pilot program offered by
the hospital where she delivered her baby. These two immigrant
women, unlike many immigrant women of color, were not referred for
a home visit in spite of their inexperience with infants and lack of
available family support. They were not labeled "knowledge deficient."
They were not labeled "at risk." What, then, are the criteria that
precipitate a home visit referral for some immigrant new mothers and
not others? It appears that if the new mother is an immigrant from
Haiti, Brazil, El Salvador, Cambodia, China, or Vietnam she will be
referred for a home visit and, often, given diagnosis of "knowledge
deficit" or "infant at risk."

Are these immigrant mothers really at high risk for negative health
outcomes? If so, why? In what ways can the health care system provide
social and emotional support to immigrant mothers?

## THE CONCEPT OF RISK: MARGINALIZATION OF MOTHERS' EXPERIENCE

The concept of risk has been widely utilized in health care for nearly
30 years. Michael Hayes (1992) conducted a Medline search in an
attempt to lend some meaning to the word and its application. He
uncovered a spectrum of topics that included the application of the
concept of risk, ranging from the perspective of evaluation and delivery
of health care to the formulation of health care policy. He identified
three spheres of literature in which the primary focus of concern is risk.
For this chapter, *health risk appraisal,* also commonly referred to as
*health risk assessment,* is the context in which the term "infant at risk"
is used. Health risk assessment was developed as a tool to assist

physicians with the prevention of disease and morbidity. The assessment attempts to identify health risk by evaluating an individual's health-related practices, habits, lifestyle, and personal characteristics as well as personal and family medical history: "Thus attributes of the individual are cast as the source of risk and the objective or intervention is to reduce the burden of premature death by stimulating individuals to stop or modify 'risky' behaviors" (Hayes, 1992, p. 402).

Even though health risk assessment is intended philosophically to be preventive, it continues to operate within a sickness model. The term "risk" is associated with negative outcomes and assigns blame or responsibility to the individual. What was implied in Claudia's referral was the potential for abuse and neglect. What was characterized as a risk, in her case, was her inability to speak English proficiently. This language barrier led to the assumption that she was uneducated and therefore lacked knowledge both in managing her own postpartum care and her baby's care. It was presumed that this knowledge deficit would jeopardize a positive health outcome for her and her baby.

In contrast to health risk assessment, the World Health Organization (WHO) utilizes the *risk approach* framework in the context of its Maternal Child Health program to maximize the efficiency of deploying resources, specifically the delivery of primary health care services. The risk approach acknowledges determinants of health that are embedded in social structure and may be beyond an individual's control, such as poverty. WHO advocates a socioecological approach to health that empowers both the individual and the community (Hayes, 1992). Within that framework, WHO would take into consideration that Claudia is without her family and a strong social community, both of which serve as a support network. WHO would support her by providing a helper who is both fluent in her language and familiar with the cultural practices related to postpartum and newborn care. Claudia would be empowered to access available community resources.

## The Use of Language and Labels

Hayes draws from D. Nelkin, who stresses how language can be used either to minimize or to maximize "risk": "Some words imply disorder or chaos, others certainty and scientific precision. Selective use of labels can trivialize an event or render it important; marginalize some groups, empower others; define an issue as a problem or reduce it to routine" (Hayes, 1992, p. 403).

The medical milieu has embraced the term "high risk" for three decades. When an individual or group is identified to be at risk, a strategy for intervention is implemented. Even if well intended, we should scrutinize the use of labels and their implications for society's view of these mothers. Are immigrant mothers at high risk for poor health outcomes? What are the sources of risks? What does it mean to be labeled "high risk"? What do we know about Brazilian, Haitian, Spanish, Asian, and Latino parenting and childrearing practices in comparison to ours?

The dominant, Eurocentric culture places a high value on independence. However, nuclear, insular families—the American model—can create isolation, stress, and loneliness. This phenomenon has an impact on all new parents arriving home with a new baby. The isolation can be intensified for immigrant mothers because of their lack of fluency in English. Their ability to access support via the telephone is dramatically impaired. A Brazilian immigrant, for example, knows that she would be tended to by a network of family and close friends if she were living in her home culture. She would not expect to know beforehand about newborn care and breastfeeding. In her homeland she would rely heavily on the advice and support of her mother and other members of her extended family. The U.S.-born mother, on the other hand, embraces the myth, perpetuated by our health care system, that because she has biologically delivered her baby she should know how to breastfeed and care for her newborn. She, compared to the immigrant mother, may be also at risk for a poor health outcome, but for different reasons.

## THE RISK:
## POOR PREGNANCY OUTCOMES

Low birthweight, a major predictor of infant mortality in the first year of life, is one example of a poor pregnancy outcome. Even though the United States is one of the wealthiest countries in the world and prides itself on advanced medical technology, in the area of infant mortality it is ranked well below other industrial nations of the world. One possible explanation for this is the continuing flow of migration into this country. Numerous studies continue to be conducted in an attempt to associate low birthweight with immigrant populations. One study, conducted by Gann, Nghiem, and Warner (1989) looked at Cambodian refugees and low-income, English-speaking white women living in

Lowell, Massachusetts. Both groups were receiving obstetrical services at the same clinic and hospital. Comparison data from low-income English-speaking white and non-Asian women participating in the statewide Maternal and Infant Care (MIC) Program were included. The study found that the prevalence of low birthweight was less in the Cambodian group than the clinic comparison and the MIC group. This investigation assessed that "contrary to our expectations prior to this study, the Cambodian refugees had more favorable birth outcomes than White low-income women in Lowell and low-income women in Massachusetts. The prevalence of low-birthweight infants, stillbirths, major pregnancy complications, and primary cesarean delivery were all lower in the Cambodian population" (Gann et al., 1989, p. 254).

A similar study in Canada was conducted in 1992 to determine if the widespread perception that immigrant mothers are at risk for adverse birth outcomes revealed similar results. The study found that there was no evidence that immigrant mothers are at higher risk of bearing low-birthweight babies or premature infants than Canadian-born mothers (Doucet, Baumgarten, & Infante-Rivard, 1992).

A comparative study between foreign-born and U.S.-born black women was conducted in 1990 to determine if there were any differences in health behaviors and birth outcomes. The study was based on the fact that black neonates are at high risk for low birthweight and perinatal mortality. The percentage of births to black foreign mothers has increased since 1976, especially in the northeast United States (Cabral, Fried, Levenson, Amaro, & Zuckerman, 1990). The results of this study also found that the incidence of low birthweight and prematurity was less for foreign-born black women, who represented Haiti, Jamaica, other Caribbean countries, Africa, Cape Verde, and England, than for U.S.-born black women (Cabral et al., 1990). In sum, most recent research has found that immigrant mothers pose a lower obstetrical risk than native-born mothers.

In an effort to understand this phenomenon, some studies have focused on the association between acculturation and the higher likelihood for a better birth outcome. Acculturation is defined as "the adoption of cultural traits, one of which is language" (Curtis, 1990, p. 148). Scribner and Dwyer (1989) explored this belief by studying Latina mothers born in Mexico compared with U.S.-born Latina mothers from the Hispanic Health and Nutrition Examination Survey. Three of the acculturation variables included language preference, ethnic identification, and nativity status. The study revealed that Latina mothers born in Mexico were less likely to have low-birthweight infants than mothers of

Mexican descent born in the United States. Mexican-born Latinas demonstrated better nutrition, fewer premarital births, and lower incidence of smoking and alcohol consumption, and possessed a higher regard for parental roles when compared to U.S.-born Mexican women (Scribner & Dwyer, 1989). To further complicate the research findings, the Mexican-born Latinas received inconsistent prenatal care. Compliance with prenatal care, that is, regular medical visits throughout the pregnancy, is considered a form of prevention for low-birthweight infants. However, visiting a health care facility when one is well is highly unusual for many immigrant groups. Pregnancy, in many other countries, is considered a normal, natural occurrence. Seeking medical assistance is reserved for identified problems during the pregnancy. Immigrant women who do not keep scheduled prenatal appointments are labeled "noncompliant" and "at risk" for a poor pregnancy outcome. "However, Mexican-born Latinos have a lower rate of low-birthweight infants than their U.S. born counterparts despite the fact they are more likely to receive late or no prenatal care" (Scribner & Dwyer, 1989, p. 1267).

Scribner and Dwyer (1989) suggest that prenatal care may be more necessary as Mexican immigrant women become more acculturated and steadily lose or give up Mexican values and beliefs, which appear to serve as a protection against low-birthweight infants. It appears that low socioeconomic status (SES) may be a stronger predictor for low-birthweight infants than origin of birth and immigrant status.

García Coll (1989) compared and contrasted United States versus Puerto Rican adolescent pregnancy and birth. She explored the social and cultural influences of adolescent pregnancy outcomes. Based on her research, SES, early prenatal care, and other health habits were more influential on the obstetric experience and perinatal outcome than age or ethnicity. Her research further suggests that SES and education are more consistently identified as determining characteristics of the caregiving environment or the developmental outcome of infants of adolescent mothers (García Coll, 1989). Her findings support the research of Belsky and colleagues (Belsky & Rovine, 1984; Belsky & Kelly, 1994), Oakley (1992), and Fraktman (1997), which stresses that a supportive environment reduces negative health outcomes for both mother and infant regardless of immigrant status. In addition, one's living conditions can pose a significant health hazard. Substandard living conditions have been found to be directly related to a rise in the number of inner city children afflicted with asthma (Malveaux & Fletcher-Vincent, 1995). A recent study, led by Dr. David Rosenstreich et al. (1997) of the Albert Einstein College of Medicine in New York found that cockroaches found in the homes of families living in impoverished neighborhoods constituted a significant allergen of asthmatic symptoms in children.

## Ana-Maria

Ana-Maria was a 30-year-old woman who immigrated to Boston from the Dominican Republic. She delivered twins in a Boston hospital. The twins were referred for skilled nursing visits due to prematurity and low birthweight. My visits took me to Ana-Maria's home, a multifamily wooden structure that was in disrepair. There were no screens on many of the windows. Ana-Maria and her twins lived in one large room in the first-floor apartment. Another mother and her young son, who suffered with asthma and was receiving home-visiting services, shared the remainder of the living space. The apartment was infested with cockroaches. Flypaper was tacked along the wall where it intersected with the ceiling. Dead cockroaches were stuck to the flypaper. When I suggested that this problem should be reported to the Board of Health, Ana-Maria was resistant. I assured her that I would assist her. She told me that if she became too vocal and too visible it would jeopardize her chances of becoming a U.S. citizen. She was adamant and could not be persuaded to change her position.

A few weeks later, during one of my visits, inspectors from the Housing Bureau came unannounced. I was quite vocal about the unacceptable living conditions. They took notes. If any action was taken, it was not apparent to me when I made subsequent visits.

This example is one of many that I encounter in my clinical practice that illustrates how immigrant mothers are exploited and marginalized. The health of this family is jeopardized by poverty and substandard living conditions. These constitute a risk to the physical and emotional health of the mother and her children. Ana-Maria's immigrant status and "knowledge deficit" does not impose a risk for her infants. The problem is, rather, that they are placed at risk by a larger system (over which they have little control).

## THE RISK: POSTPARTUM DEPRESSION

Stern and Kruckman (1983) believe that postpartum depression in the United States may represent a culture-bound syndrome. Their premise is based on observations of the birthing and postpartum experience in other cultures as well as the review of cross-cultural literature, which reveals little evidence of postpartum depression. They believe that postpartum depression in nonpsychotic forms is exacerbated by the lack of sociocultural structuring of the postpartum period in this country. Elements often observed in other countries/cultures include protective measures such as social seclusion, mandated rest, and assistance with household tasks from family and/or midwives. These measures reflect the vulnerability of the new mother and her need for support especially in the immediate postpartum period. The authors observed rituals that represented both the social status of becoming a mother and assistance in the process of reentering the social community in that new role.

The immigrant mother often lacks a family support network, cultural rituals, and a social community. We, as health care providers, have been unconscious of the isolation created by the arrangement of nuclear family units. Sonia is an example.

### Sonia

Sonia was a 32-year-old Portuguese-speaking Brazilian woman who had delivered her first baby. She had sustained a third-degree vaginal laceration in the delivery process. She wanted to breastfeed her baby. She had no family members in this country. Her partner worked out of state for long periods of time. He was preparing to leave and would not return for 1 month. Her health insurance approved only two home visits. The visiting nurse, who made the initial visit, spoke no Portuguese. Without additional approved visits there was a high likelihood that this woman would develop postpartum depression. But in order to advocate for additional visits the "patient" must look sick. Our health care system, which advertises preventative medicine, is driven by economics and pathology. The notion of postpartum support provided by trained professionals and lay persons is viewed as costly and not necessary. The American health care system frequently discounts and challenges medical assessments in order to keep costs down. This health care system, in fact, *contributes* to placing this woman, and many like her, *at risk* for postpartum depression. Ours is a country that is more willing to spend its money on research to determine the cause for the rising incidence of postpartum depression than on providing social support to prevent it. The health care system throws the safety net after the fall rather than providing a fabric of preventive community support.

Postpartum depression is not unique to immigrant women. Rather, it is a phenomenon that is experienced by all too many women in the immediate postpartum period. It is compounded, however, for the immigrant mother, who lacks the family and community to provide support. Her inability to speak the language limits her ability to access help, which increases her isolation.

The severity of the laceration, the discernible fatigue of this new mother, and the difficulties she was experiencing as she attempted to breastfeed her baby were arguments by the visiting nurse that were strong enough to persuade the health insurance reviewer to approve an additional visit.

The process of immigration can thus put added stress on a woman's adjustment to her new role as a mother. As such, although not at risk for negative birth outcomes, immigrant mothers might be at a higher risk for postpartum depression.

## IMMIGRATION AS A PROCESS

The process of immigration and resettling is disequilibriating and stress provoking. Often family and community support is absent. In an American nuclear family model, mothers, at home with young children, become even more isolated. This can lead to further debilitation and possible depression. Monica McGoldrick (1982) stresses the disruptive nature of migration: "The readjustment to a new culture is by no means a single event, it is a prolonged developmental process of adjustment, which will affect family members differently, depending on the life cycle phase they are in at the time of the transition" (McGoldrick, 1982, p. 17). She suggests that families who must negotiate the immigration process add an extra life stage to their life cycle.

Often the impetus to leave one's place of origin is the hope of improving one's life with the expectation of having greater opportunities to fulfill one's own personal dreams. Pollock (1989) refers to this particular form of leave-taking as "voluntary migration." He notes that "despite the voluntary aspect of this venturing, there still are elements of mourning, loss, nostalgia, memories and feelings of the past that are positive as well as negative" (p. 145). Others leave their homeland for political asylum and personal safety. Their sense of loss should not be underestimated. Angelina is an example.

### Angelina

Angelina, 22, left El Salvador 9 years ago with her father and older brother. Throughout her adolescence her father's overprotective behavior prevented her from developing any friendships. At age 17, she met a boy, and moved in with him. She referred to him as her boyfriend. At age 22, she delivered a baby girl, and 7 weeks later our agency received a referral to evaluate Angelina for postpartum depression. As I gathered information about her family, the lack of information she shared regarding her mother was striking. When I asked about her mother her expression changed dramatically. She appeared sad and close to tears. She responded, "That's the missing piece." I asked for clarification. She told me that her mother still lived in El Salvador and did not want to come to the United States. She had not seen her mother since she left El Salvador nine years before. It was too expensive for her to visit her mother, or even to phone her. Angelina said that she had written her mother, but for some unexplained reason her mother never received the letters. Quietly and sadly she remarked, "I write all my feelings in the letters and the feelings get lost." Angelina said that she had experienced sadness over the past 9 years whenever she thought about her mother. She thought she had overcome those feelings; however, having the baby reawakened memories of her mother and her experience as a daughter.

Psychotherapist Joyce Block, PhD, suggests that assuming the role of mother often forces a woman to revise her relationship with her own mother: "The experience of caring for a baby stirs up early memories and sensations for all and reminds each woman that she was once as helpless and dependent as her baby is now" (Block, 1990, p. 21). Author Jane Swigart concurs. She suggests that a new mother often reexperiences the longings she once had for her own mother as she attempts to respond to her own infant's dependency needs (Swigart, 1991). Angelina's profound sadness about missing her mother supports McGoldrick's (1982) premise that immigration is a prolonged developmental process that impacts on events in one's life cycle at different times. Could Angelina's postpartum depression have been prevented? I believe that if health care professionals spent as much time gathering a family history as they do gathering medical history, Angelina's unresolved sad feelings in leaving her mother were more likely to have been detected earlier. Had this been the case, opportunities to help Angelina express her feelings could have begun during her pregnancy. By taking the time to listen to Angelina's story, the health care provider could have initiated a process to help her access support during this major life transition. It would have been an opportunity to assist her in the work of grieving the loss of her mother as she prepared to become a mother herself.

Angelina recounted meeting two women in the hospital clinic waiting room. One woman had a 5-month-old baby, and the other was pregnant. Angelina stated:

"Just on an impulse I asked them for their telephone number. I thought maybe we could visit one another. I've never done anything like that. I guess I was desperate."

Health care workers trained to think within the terms of traditional health risk assessment may underestimate the sadness, sense of loss, and unresolved grief experienced by immigrants. Their need to mourn is trivialized.

## NEWLY ARRIVED IMMIGRANTS FROM BRAZIL

In 1993, I conducted an independent research study. The purpose of that study was to examine the childbearing and childrearing practices of recently arrived immigrant mothers from Brazil. All the participants spoke of the difficulties they experienced as they attempted to adjust, with the New England weather just one of many new challenges. That seemingly minor adjustment, however, went beyond the cold and snow. It included deprivation of light, multiple layers of clothing that they found restrictive, and, most significantly, confinement indoors, which pointed up the lack of family and community. One mother who had just delivered her first baby remarked:

"The days are so short. You have long nights. That's a kind of depression, because you have a lot of time to think about your family and friends and miss them."

To resist the isolation, she surrounded herself with photographs of her family. In this context she described the living arrangements she left behind in Brazil. She told me that she was one of six children, the "baby" in the family. As she talked about her family and introduced me to them by way of photographs, her expression saddened. She confided, "I miss my family. I miss my mother."

Rosa succinctly shed light on why new mothers in the early postpartum period don't receive help from other Brazilian women in America:

"In America everybody do a lot. They don't have time. Just a quick visit and that's it. In America all the people are working a lot. No time for help anybody."

One mother confided that being confined to the home during the winter months was a loss of freedom, that it was a dramatic loss to be unable to go outside to socialize.

The deprivation appeared to me more like a loss of spirit. Christina said:

"The worse thing is to stay home during the winter or to go to places like disco that are closed, not open. [In Brazil] if you talk to someone, you don't have to stay home to talk. You can go out. They have a lot of open places to talk, to play. But here, if you go outside, you don't stay long outside. You don't do barbecues, you don't go to beaches. And if you go outside, you use hat and gloves. We don't do that."

The persistent longing for the family was also impressive. It is customary in other cultures, including Brazil, that childcare responsibilities are shared by extended family members. These Brazilian women who delivered their babies in the United States were deeply saddened that their families, especially their mothers, were not with them. This absence was clearly a void for these new mothers. They had relied heavily on support and direction from their mothers and extended family. This cultural practice, which is eroded by the immigration process, accentuates the sadness and longing for family members, especially after the birth of a baby (Hattar-Pollara & Meleis, 1995). The yearning for family and friends was compounded for some by their children who desperately wanted to return to Brazil. Tania is an example.

### Tania

When I met Tania she had been in this country only 4 months. She and her two children had recently arrived from Brazil to be with her husband, who was studying at a local university. She confided that this was her first trip outside of Brazil. In fact, she confessed that she had never traveled outside of her small community. She repeatedly told me how hard it was for her to adjust. "I don't know many people here. I go to the supermarket, and then I go home." As I continued the interview she repeated:

"I don't have friends. I don't have my family. It's not my country. It's different. In Brazil, I lived with my mom. Near my house is the house of my uncle. I had a lot of friends."

Her facial expression changed. Tears began to roll down her cheeks. She denied she was sad. She said:

"I'm not sad, I'm not sad. Just remembering my life in Brazil. It is most difficult because my youngest son is sad all day. He says all the time, 'Mom, I want to go back to Brazil!' "

Her own sadness was compounded by her son's grief. In contrast, a parent's own grieving and anxiety reaction can impact on available supportive efforts that are directed toward the children (García Coll & Magnuson, 1997). Tania's compromised ability to speak English, the adjustment to unfamiliar surroundings and climate increased her loneliness and longing, like that of her son, to return home.

## RESISTING HIGH-RISK LABELS: SUPPORT, ADVOCACY, AND COLLABORATION

What are some ways that the health care system can facilitate a smoother transition for immigrant mothers? Universal postpartum support is one viable solution that can facilitate a smoother transition for immigrant mothers in the immediate and early postpartum period. By virtue of being universal, this support implies no stigma, no emergency, and no abnormality (Wharf, 1988). Universal support acknowledges that transitioning into the parenting role is stress provoking for all new parents. It acknowledges that parenting is hard work. Transitioning to the parenting role and the hard work of parenting warrant some degree of postpartum support.

Vaux (1988) suggests that there are three major functions of social support: (1) It should provide supplementary assistance, (2) it should sustain feelings of being cared for and valued, and (3) it should sustain a sense of social identity and social location. He stresses the importance of protecting and nurturing autonomy without undermining efficacy.

Support is directed toward acknowledging the recipient's strengths and empowering her or him to explore available support networks. Advocacy is a form of support: "If support is related to disorder directly, then a case could be made for promoting support among the general population, not just those at high risk for stressors. If support is seen as meeting basic social needs, promoting it among only high risk groups might ignore the majority of potential beneficiaries" (Vaux, 1988, p. 243).

Research has identified that immigrant women who are isolated and experience cultural tension within the family can develop a range of social and psychological problems including extreme unhappiness, psychosomatic disorders, neurosis, and even psychotic disorders (Hattar-Pollara & Meleis, 1995).

Health care professionals can help to mediate some of these maladies. They can learn to be open to developing a better understanding of immigrant mothers' experiences of negotiating a new culture while attempting to maintain their own cultural integrity. Asking the individual what she would do if she were in her home culture conveys interest and a sensitive understanding that can enhance informed participation. Health care professionals can assist immigrant mothers by providing emotional support. Health care providers need to resist the messages of a Eurocentric medical system, and when feasible they can assist immigrant mothers in accessing similar ethnic groups. "Ethnic groups can facilitate immigrants' adaptation and contribute to their psychological well-being by buffering or preventing the stress associated with immigration" (Hattar-Pollara & Meleis, 1995, p. 208).

## COLLABORATING, NEGOTIATING, AND EMPOWERING IMMIGRANT MOTHERS

Hernandez (1995) suggests that immigration is only the point of entry. The new immigrant faces marginalization, and her status may be subject to change. She is without community, thus support. Hernandez stresses that acculturation is a negotiation of two cultures. In what ways can we, in the helping professions, assist in this negotiation process? Hernandez says it can be done through empowerment.

Eliana Korin (1995), coordinator of the residency program at Montefiore Medical Center in Bronx, New York, describes the barriers to empowerment: discrimination, a reduction of support networks, chronic stress, helplessness and hopelessness, long-term poverty, and perceived inability. We in the health care system can actively help to break down those barriers. We can negotiate and collaborate with immigrant mothers.

### Suna

Suna was a 28-year-old woman from Afghanistan. She was referred with the diagnosis of knowledge deficit and infant at risk after the birth of her second child. She was breastfeeding her baby. On my third visit to her home she expressed a concern. She told me that she didn't have enough milk. She added that her milk wasn't "strong enough." I asked her how she knew. She told me that she didn't think her baby was satisfied. "She cries," she told me. I asked her if she had breastfed her first child. She acknowledged that she had. "But," she said, "he was born in my country. If I were in my country the women would bring me sugar cane." She told me that eating the sugar cane and drinking its freshly squeezed, sweet juice would make her milk strong and help increase the volume of milk. She was certain that these two conditions would satisfy her baby. She confided, "My husband told me that I would have to find out where I could get some. I can't use the telephone. It is too hard for me. People talk too fast."

I began making inquiries. I placed a call to a local Japanese market. They suggested that I try Chinatown. I pondered. The Amazon. Brazil! I placed a call to the Brazilian/American Language Institute. I spoke with my friend and codirector. "Yes," she said, "I have heard that sugar cane helps improve a mother's milk. The market across the street sells sugar cane." She gave me the number and the name of the proprietor, who said, "We have a fresh supply of sugar cane every 3 days. We have fresh squeezed sugar cane juice daily." Suna was grateful. When I returned the following week she told me that she has been eating sugar cane and drinking the sugar cane juice. She smiled and said, "My baby is satisfied."

Providing health care goes beyond rendering a health assessment. Speaking the native language helps, but it is not enough. The health care professional must respect a belief system that may not be familiar or congruent with her or his own. One must be open and receptive to another way of thinking or different health care practices. This is collaborating with the client and respecting differences rather than labeling them as risks. It empowers the woman by supporting and respecting her belief system, her health care practices, and her language.

## AN ENGLISH-ONLY POLICY

The demand for an English-only policy has resurfaced in the political arena. If enacted, it would directly impact on the collaboration and empowerment of immigrant mothers. English only as a policy is not new. Before the American Revolution, Benjamin Franklin worried that the Pennsylvania colony would be governed in German, ultimately requiring the services of interpreters in the Assembly. Some English-only laws began to appear as the influx of immigrants in the mid-1800s posed a threat to the dominant Puritan group, but at the turn of the 20th century many schools taught in the native language of the students. U.S. immigration laws in the 1940s and 1950s required English proficiency to enter this country, but there were major changes in immigration policies and a favoring of bilingual education in the 1960's. The trend to support such programs and policies began to diminish in the 1980s. "A backlash against the perceived 'excessive' gains of minorities at the expense of the white majority became a strident vocal opposition to non-English instruction in the classroom and non-English languages in government documents" (Brown, 1992, p. 10).

In 1988, an Arizona state constitutional amendment was narrowly approved that would have imposed the toughest of the nation's growing number of English-only language restrictions. However, the amendment was argued before the Supreme Court and struck down. Supporters of an English-only policy believe that exclusive use of English would speed up the assimilation process, help unify an ethnically diverse nation, and help to make government more efficient. Opponents cite the history, which has demonstrated that restrictive language policies inspire resistance and discord ("English-Only Faces," 1996). My experience is that access to native speakers is much more helpful to assimilation than not.

### Esmeira

Esmeira was a 30-year-old Somalian woman who was referred with a diagnosis of knowledge deficit after she delivered her third child. I visited her regularly over 4 months. Initially the visits required an interpreter. Esmeira was enrolled in a GED program. Over the course of those 4 months, there were noticeable changes in her. As she developed more facility expressing herself in English, she more readily articulated her concerns and feelings. She openly told of past abuses from her estranged husband that she and her children experienced. She became more animated during the visits. She asked me to assist her making telephone calls. She desired to have a better command of English so she could find employment. I believe an English-only policy might have prevented or at the very least retarded this interactive process.

In the late 1970s only one hospital in the greater Boston area provided written materials and signage in a language other than English. The use of paid professional interpreters was rare. In the early 1980s the son of an elderly Greek-speaking woman was not allowed to be with his mother in the recovery room to help orient her as she emerged from anesthesia. Rather, an employee from the housekeeping department, a total stranger, was expected to "translate," if it was necessary. In the 1990s there is a movement in the health care industry, albeit a slow one, that has begun to respond to the linguistic and cultural differences of its consumers. The notion that paid interpreters are too costly an expenditure has gradually begun to change.

I believe that some of the change is demonstrated by how clients access health care services. Because neighborhood clinics often provide native-speaking staff, and are closer and easier to access, immigrant mothers are utilizing these clinics for prenatal, postpartum, and pediatric services. The keen competition for clients among hospitals may thus be an impetus for change. In fact, immigrant women who require obstetrical services seem to have motivated some hospitals to employ bilingual staff.

An English-only policy would eliminate such services. It would create isolation, especially for mothers who remain at home with young children. It would accentuate their difference and contribute to the negative labels of "high risk" and "knowledge deficit." We could begin to see unmet health care appointments, which will be interpreted as noncompliance. The efforts of native-speaking health care professionals, who have informed clients of appropriate access to care, will be eradicated. The use of the emergency room for health care needs, which is a costly mode of health care practice, will begin to increase.

An English-only policy is disempowering. It is a ploy by the white dominant culture to maintain control and power.

Rather than assigning blame to immigrant mothers who do not speak English, we, as a society, need to ask what provisions are made available to them to foster and encourage them to learn English. Unlike other countries such as Canada, Israel, and Australia, the U.S. government has a laissez-faire immigrant policy that places the resettlement and integration responsibility on state and local government. Funding for such programs has declined. The attitude that supports this lack of interest is not new. It is based on the assumption that most immigrants are self-sufficient and are not the government's responsibility (Fix & Zimmerman, 1997). Thus, immigrant mothers who may be motivated to learn English have very limited resources to do so. Health care providers need to resist the English-only movement and advocate on behalf of motivated families.

## CONCLUSION

I have attempted to examine the notion of "high risk" and how its present use marginalizes immigrant mothers. The use of this labeling creates stereotyping, accentuates differences, and interprets them as deficits. Lack of sensitivity to immigrants' culture can contribute to isolation, which can lead to physical and psychological disturbances. Our present health care system, with its emphasis on pathology and crisis, contributes to discriminatory labeling practices, which help to marginalize immigrant mothers. The threat of an English-only policy could create a major setback in how the host culture interacts with this group, contributing to their further alienation.

Health care professionals have an opportunity to be leaders in effecting change on behalf of immigrant mothers. Presenting at conferences, dispelling stereotypes by sharing accurate information in the workplace, encouraging the implementation of interpretive services, and collaborating with immigrant mothers are some examples of assuming a leadership role. Health care professionals as a lobbying group can impact the political arena on issues such as an English-only policy and services for legal immigrants.

Immigrant mothers share the same hopes, desires, and deep caring for their children and families as their U.S.-born counterparts. They are strong. Many have experienced oppression, deprivation, and violence in their homeland. Most come with the hope of a better life. They bring a cultural richness that they, with little provocation, are eager to share. That cultural richness contributes to the fabric of this country.

Like a woven tapestry, its beauty lies in its variety of colors and its strength in the overlapping fibers.

## REFERENCES

Belsky, J., & Kelly, J. (1994). *The transition to parenthood.* New York: Delacorte Press.

Belsky, J., & Rovine, M. (1984, May). Social-network contact, family support and the transition to parenthood. *Journal of Marriage and the Family,* 455–462.

Blackburn, S. T. (1992). *Maternal, fetal and neonatal physiology: A clinical perspective.* Philadelphia: Saunders.

Block, J. (1990). *Motherhood as metamorphosis.* New York: Plume.

Brown, B. (1992). *The history of bilingual education in America* (Educational Document 350874). Washington, DC: U.S. Department of Education Office of Educational Research and Improvement.

Cabral, H., Fried, L., Levenson, S., Amaro, H., & Zuckerman, B. (1990). Foreign born and US born black women: Differences in health behaviors and birth outcomes. *American Journal of Public Health, 80,* 70–72.

Curtis, P. A. (1990). The consequences of acculturation to service delivery and research with Hispanic families. *Child and Social Work, 7,* 147–159.

Doucet, H., Baumgarten, M., & Infante-Rivard, C. (1992). Risk of low birthweight and prematurity among foreign born mothers. *Canadian Journal of Public Health, 83*(3), 192–195.

English-only faces free speech test. (1996, November 28). *The Boston Globe,* p. B28.

Ewy, D. H., & Youmans, J. (1988). The early parenting experience. In F. Nichols & S. Humenick (Eds.), *Childbirth education: Practice, research and theory.* Philadelphia: Saunders.

Fix, M., & Zimmerman, W. (1997). Immigrant families and public policy: A deepening divide. In A. Booth, A. Crouter, & N. Landale (Eds.), *Immigration and the family.* Mahwah, NJ: Erlbaum.

Fraktman, M. (1993). *Parenting: A cultural perspective.* Unpublished independent study, Lesley College, Cambridge, MA.

Fraktman, M. (1997). *Determining the degree of needed support in the immediate and early postpartum period.* Unpublished doctoral dissertation, Lesley College, Cambridge, MA.

Gann, P., Nghiem, L., & Warner, S. (1989). Pregnancy characteristics and outcomes of Cambodian refugees. *American Journal of Public Health, 79*(9), 1251–1257.

García Coll, C. (1989). The consequences of teenage childbearing in traditional Puerto Rican culture. In K. Nugent, B. Lester, & T. Brazelton (Eds.), *The cultural context of infancy.* Norwood, NJ: Ablex.

García Coll, C., & Magnuson, K. (1997). The psychological experience of immigration: A developmental perspective. In A. Booth, A. Crouter, & N. Landale (Eds.), *Immigration and the family.* Mahwah, NJ: Erlbaum.

Gladieux, J. D. (1978). The transition to parenthood: Satisfaction with the pregnancy experience as a function of sex role conceptions, marital relationship, and social network. In W. B. Miller & L. Newman (Eds.), *The first child and family formation.* Chapel Hill, NC: University of North Carolina at Chapel Hill Press.

Hattar-Pollara, M., & Meleis, A. I. (1995). Parenting their adolescents: The experiences of Jordanian immigrant women in California. *Healthcare for Women International, 16,* 195–211.

Hayes, M. (1992). On the epistemology of risk: Language, logic and social science. *Social Science and Medicine, 35*(4), 401–407.

Hernandez, M. (1995, June). *Listening to narratives of refugees and immigrants from various cultures.* Paper presented at the AFTA symposium, "Clinical Dimensions of Migration, Immigration, Culture and Class," Cambridge, MA.

Korin, E. (1995, June). *Applying Paolo Freire's liberational approach to clinical work with migrants, immigrants and refugees.* Presentation at the AFTA symposium, "Clinical Dimensions of Migration, Immigration, Culture and Class," Cambridge, MA.

Malveaux, F. J., & Fletcher-Vincent, S. A. (1995). Environmental risk factors of childhood asthma in urban centers. *Environmental Health Perspectives, 6,* 59–62.

McGoldrick, M. (1982). Ethnicity and family therapy: An overview. In M. McGoldrick, J. K. Pearce, & J. Giordano (Eds.), *Ethnicity and family therapy* (pp. 3–30). New York: Guilford Press.

McGoldrick, M., Pearce, J. K., & Gioradano, J. (Eds.). (1982). *Ethnicity and family therapy.* New York: Guilford Press.

Mammen, O. (1993). On treating mothers with babies. *Developments, 2*(4), 2–4.

Oakley, A. (1992). *Social support and motherhood.* Cambridge, UK: Blackwell.

Plutzik, R., & Laghi, M. (1983). *The private life of parents.* New York: Everest House.

Pollock, G. (1989). On migration: Voluntary and coerced. *Annal of Psychoanalysis, 17,* 145–158.

Rose, M., & Ginnetty, K. (1989). Madonnas in mourning. *Networker,* 28–29.

Rosenstreich, D., Eggleston, P., Kattan, M., Baker, D., Slavin, R., Gergen, P., Mitchell, H., McNiff-Mortimer, K., Lynn, H., Ownby, D., & Malveaux, F. (1997). The role of cockroach allergy and exposure to cockroach allergen in causing morbidity among inner-city children with asthma. *New England Journal of Medicine, 336,* 1356–1363.

Scribner, R., & Dwyer, J. (1989). Acculturation and low birthweight among Latinos in the Hispanic Hanes. *American Journal of Public Health, 79*(9), 1263–1267.

Stern, G., & Kruckman, L. (1983). Multi-disciplinary perspectives on post-partum depression: An anthropological critique. *Social Science and Medicine, 17*(15), 1027–1041.

Swigart, J. (1991). *The myth of the bad mother: Emotional realities of mothering.* New York: Doubleday.

Vaux, A. (1988). *Social support: Theory, research and intervention.* New York: Praeger.

Weingarten, K., & Daniels, P. (1983). *Sooner or later: The timing of parenthood in adult lives.* New York: Norton.

Wharf, B. (1988). Implementing the ecological perspective in policy and practice: Problems and prospects. In A. Pence (Ed.), *Ecological research with children and families.* New York: Teachers College Press.

# *Conversation One*

*Edited by*

KATHY WEINGARTEN

A LL mothers experience marginalization, although the sources of the marginalization and the resources for mobilizing a response to it will vary significantly. In the conversation that follows we, editors and contributors, try to identify points of convergence among the preceding four groups of mothers. This conversation, like the other two in this book, has been edited down from a 2-hour discussion. Wendy Quiñones, herself the mother of an adolescent, speaks first.

WENDY QUIÑONES: At the point at which a child becomes an adolescent, society doesn't think mothers should be mothering anymore. This is one of the dilemmas that seems central to the mothers of adolescents.

KATHY WEINGARTEN: I agree. There is a socially constructed bind. It seems that the mother of the adolescent is asked to mother in a very particular way. She should be the provider (e.g., stock the refrigerator), but she is not supposed to be there when the goods are consumed. There for the work, not the play. The qualities that are valued in the mother of a young child are no longer valued in the mother of a teen.

JANET L. SURREY: What about differences of race and class?

KATHY WEINGARTEN: I am talking about mainstream, Western, probably only North American culture. If we take a racial or ethnic perspective or if we consider mothering an adolescent with special needs, the dynamics might change considerably.

ELIZABETH SPARKS: Kathy, how does resistance work for mothers of adolescents?

KATHY WEINGARTEN: One form of resistance available to any mother of an adolescent is to challenge the idea that you are passé in your adolescent's life. Intense propaganda is directed at adolescents to separate and to make the mother less central in their lives. Can you think of advertisements that show mothers and their teen children together? Moms of teens are rendered invisible. Mothers, and people who care about adolescents, can increase awareness of the push to make the mothers' importance invisible in a young person's life. We need to emphasize that there is still an essential role for the mother of adolescent to play.

WENDY QUINONES: Mothers of special needs/exceptional children get messages they must resist also. A clear message that moms get is: "If you have a child like this, then you did something wrong. Don't bother us; take care of it yourself." That message has to be resisted to stay sane.

MIRIAM GREENSPAN: I don't think the message is "You *did* something wrong." I think it is more global and devastating, more like "You are wrong. Your child is defective, and so are you."

JANET L. SURREY: I agree that, one way or the other, most moms do get the message that *they* are wrong. That may lead them to think that they have to change themselves. But it's important not to put all the expectation of resistance on individual mothers, and important not to marginalize or blame them if they don't do it. Schools, medical settings, clinical settings, and others who are involved must themselves resist and help mothers resist devaluing messages.

MARY LEWIS: One of the ways we at Wellspring help homeless mothers resist devaluing messages is to help them distinguish financial poverty, often associated with homelessness, from other problems. We try to help them see that poverty and homelessness are not a direct result of individual dysfunctions. People have problems whether they have a home or not. Financial difficulties are human problems that all people share. This helps the women form bonds with each other so they are able to take on the opposition to their devaluation as a group; they face it together.

JANET L. SURREY: In Marilyn's chapter on immigrant mothers, she aligns herself with the mothers so that together they can resist the devaluing messages. I think that her chapter speaks to the importance of resisting some of the standard practices of one's own profession by aligning with the client. Clients then experience the relationship as a safe place.

MARILYN G. FRAKTMAN: I do align with clients, and I show this in a number of ways. For instance, I make an effort to speak their language. They are so excited about my speaking their language that they correct me when I speak. There is a joining through language, and it shows mutual respect.

JANET L. SURREY: It is a wonderful way to demonstrate respect for them and their culture; it's meeting them halfway.

CYNTHIA GARCÍA COLL: Let me raise this question: Is "aligning with" significantly different from "helping those folks"? There is a danger of being condescending and marginalizing: "We will teach them [immigrants] right, this time." But what do they need to be taught? Immigrants know their experience is directly linked to issues of poverty. At the same time, immigration can be a traumatic experience with great loss and disconnection from familiar ties. Actually, homeless women and immigrant mothers both experience profound disconnection.

MARY LEWIS: I agree that loss is a significant aspect of the experience of homeless mothers, and I see some other factors as well. When I lived overseas, I worked with people who were expatriates. These people were very privileged. They had no financial problems, and yet they too were dealing with issues of isolation, of being marginalized from the dominant culture in which they now lived. They felt frustrated and helpless. The pain of isolation or feeling disconnected definitely changes people, and poverty magnifies it all.

BETSY SMITH: The institutions that interact with immigrant mothers magnify the pain too. They can be very threatening. Immigrant mothers are trying to care for their children, be accountable for them to these institutions, while they have language and other barriers. Homeless mothers live with many of the same fears and anxieties.

MARY LEWIS: Yes, the homeless women are anxious about children being removed from them. If you are a homeless mom with an adolescent son, some of the shelters won't take you in.

ELIZABETH SPARKS: We could take the themes of isolation and invisibility and find them with most of the mothers we've discussed. When people feel unacknowledged, loss exists right away. The mothers of adolescents are rendered invisible. Mothers of adolescents are "asked" to be a certain way with their children and with that comes loss. Mothers of adolescents can be maligned by society or their own children. If you don't fit societal ideas, the message often given is that you, as a mother, need treatment. When we turn our sights to mothers with special-needs children, we see isolation and invisibility as well.

CYNTHIA GARCÍA COLL: I have another parallel, between immigrant moms and mothers of adolescents. In both cases the mother simply continues "mothering" as before but suddenly it is "out of context." What was okay and customary before, now is perceived as being wrong.

REBECCA KOCH: This applies to homeless mothers as well. You are going along, in survival mode, but feeling okay about your mothering. Then suddenly circumstances arise, whatever money there was, is no longer there. You are catapulted into homelessness. Suddenly you are mothering in a very different situation and context.

KATHY WEINGARTEN: This could be described as a phenomenon of a transitory state. The immigrant mother is "in transition" by virtue of a change of country, a change in context. The homeless mother is "in transition" also because of a change in context. The mother of an adolescent is "in transition" because her child enters a particular life stage.

ELIZABETH SPARKS: The phenomenon of transition applies even in the case of mothers of children with special needs. During the pregnancy, the mother expects a healthy child. At some point, that changes, whether it is prebirth, at birth, or later. The change occurs, and a transition happens, based on the needs of the child.

WENDY QUIÑONES: There are also differences with homelessness. For some, homelessness can be an event that happened and is over, not a transition to a permanent state. When one is the mother of a special-needs child, by contrast, that is always who you are and who you remain.

MIRIAM GREENSPAN: Mothering a child with disabilities is permanent mothering. The general cultural ideas about separation, which are always problematic, are particularly so for children who have needs that are always going to keep them partially dependent on others.

KATHY WEINGARTEN: Children with special needs may be dependent on their mothers, their parents, but as Miriam points out in her chapter there is also mutuality. Miriam describes learning from Esther. She acknowledges this mutuality; that they are teacher and learner, each with the other. I see a connection with the ideas in the chapter on homeless mothers. Homeless mothers need relationships with workers that are more mutual. Staff and mothers can view motherhood as a common thread between them, regardless of who has a home and who doesn't.

MARY LEWIS: I think I can extend that thought. All the mothers would do better with relationships that are more mutual, especially those with caregivers. If you have a special-needs child, if you are new to this country, you would benefit from a caregiver working in a side-by-side position, rather than in an up–down position.

MARILYN G. FRAKTMAN: In immigrant communities, women honor their mothers as resources, as people who are in that side-by-side position. They expect their mothers to teach them by modeling alongside them. If their mothers are not in the United States, they still want their mothers to teach them. In some ways, I view myself as a surrogate.

JANET L. SURREY: Many immigrants retain the attachment to intergenerational bonds. In this culture, there seems to be a devaluing of these bonds. Individualism, and therefore isolation, are created. Also, the culture tells us that family is "exclusive." This results in a loss of community and a lack of support for mothers. For so many, there is a dangerous and devastating lack of a communal net to "hold" mothers through hardship, suffering, transition, or "special" needs. That is what we must work for.

# 5

## Yes, I Am a Swan
### Reflections on Families Headed by Lesbians and Gay Men

*LAURA BENKOV*

### THE SOCIAL CONTEXT OF LESBIAN AND GAY FAMILY FORMATION

On December 3, 1996, Judge Kevin S. C. Chang of Hawaii's First Circuit Court found that the denial of marriage licenses to gay and lesbian couples constituted gender discrimination and therefore violated the Hawaiian state constitution's guarantee to all citizens of equal protection under the law. This finding was based on his observation that the state had not proved it had a compelling interest in banning same-sex marriages. Though the state immediately appealed, thus leaving the Hawaii Supreme Court to make a final ruling on the matter, it is highly likely that that ruling will support Judge Chang's decision, because back in 1993 the Hawaii Supreme Court itself had made a similar finding (Kunen, 1996, pp. 44–45).

As I sat at my kitchen table reading Judge Chang's decision, my not quite 3-year-old daughter, Elizabeth, and her slightly younger friend, Amy, were animatedly dancing a few feet away from me, announcing joyfully that they were getting married. "Having a wedding" was one of Elizabeth's favorite games of the moment. Sometimes she married Amy, sometimes her little cousin Joshua, and sometimes, when she was feeling particularly warmly toward me, I got to be the lucky bride. To Elizabeth weddings have something to do with love, but more importantly at the moment, something to do with music, dress up, dance, and celebration.

Although 2 months younger than Elizabeth, her cousin Joshua is somewhat farther along in knowing the real rules of the game. He got his first lesson a short time ago from an old family friend. Exuberantly he declared his intention to marry Elizabeth, but he was quickly told that because she is his cousin that would not be possible. Though momentarily disappointed, he easily rallied, deciding instead to marry his best friend, Harry. Alas, he was told that too would not do—couldn't he think of a nice little girl to marry? Stymied at first, eventually he came up with the name of an acquaintance who fit the bill—unrelated and the right gender.

The story was recounted to me with some chagrin by my sister who lamented the fact that she hadn't acted on her impulse to tell Joshua that his wish to marry Harry was just fine. Adding to the significance of the story in our family context was the fact that the friend who'd suggested that Joshua think of a nice girl to marry had been and continues to be one of our extended family members who is most supportive of my alternative family structure. She was the first to embrace my union with a woman, and she lovingly rejoiced in the birth of my daughter, conceived through donor insemination when I was single. I doubt that she experiences any contradiction between her admonishments to Joshua and her loving support of Elizabeth and me.

Upon hearing the story I thought this is how the idealization of heterosexual procreative unions and the concomitant marginalization of all other family forms gains such a stronghold on our psyches. The messages come to the very young both from those who know and love them well and, via the media, from those who don't know them at all. The statements are tautological and presented matter of factly as self-evident. But increasingly, children like Joshua and Elizabeth, whose own families contain myriad configurations that work well, must sort through contradictory messages. Theirs will be the consciousness of the future.

Reading Judge Chang's decision with the sound of Elizabeth's and Amy's delighted squealing in the background brought Joshua to mind. His uncomprehending acquiescence to the rules of heterosexuality, a private act, bears strong resemblance to the public discourse surrounding the roles of lesbians and gay men in family life. Vehemently held claims that homosexuality exists in opposition to family life and that gay men and lesbians are dangerous to children surface repeatedly, their impact scarcely affected by the degree to which they are unsubstantiated. Given this context, I agree with Evan Wolfson, co-counsel for the three couples, who declared that Judge Chang's decision marks an "extraordinary turning point" (Kunen, 1996, p. 44). Not only did it set the stage for applying gender discrimination ruling in other cases, but it also urged people to eschew the fetishization of the so-called "traditional" heterosexual, procreative, legally sanctioned family unit in favor of a true embracing of diverse family forms imbued with the recognition that it is the quality of our relationships rather than the structure of our families that matters most in human development.

The Hawaii decision was significant not because of its pragmatic value, which is limited, but rather, because of the extent to which Judge Chang challenged knee-jerk homophobic assumptions, insisting instead that a deeper level of thought prevail. Specifically, Judge Chang noted that the state failed to "prove that the public interest in the well-being of children and families, or the optimal development of children will be adversely affected by same-sex marriage" (*Baehr v. Miike,* 1996). He based that finding largely on two aspects of the testimony he had heard. One was the increasing body of psychological literature demonstrating that children raised by lesbian and/or gay parents are virtually indistinguishable from children raised by heterosexual parents in all aspects of their development (Hoeffer, 1981; Kirkpatrick, Smith, & Roy, 1981; Kweskin & Cook, 1982; Miller, Jacobsen, & Bigner, 1981; Pagelow, 1980; Patterson, 1992; Rand, Graham, & Rawlings, 1982).The other was a basic but often overlooked point made by a psychologist who provided expert testimony. Dr. David Brodzinsky of Rutgers University noted:

> The issue is not the structural variable: biological versus nonbiological, one parent versus two parents. They hide, I think, what's really going on. The issue is really the process variables: how children are cared for, is the child provided warmth, is the child provided consistency of care, is the child provided a stimulating environment, is the child given support. Those are the factors we can call, for lack of a better way of saying it, sensitive care-giving, which transcend whether you're a single parent, two parent, biological, or nonbiological parent. The research shows that those are the factors that carry the biggest weight. And when you look at structural variables there's not all that much support that they are in and of themselves all that important. (*Baehr v. Miike,* 1996, p. 29).

Dr. Brodzinsky went on to explain his presence as a child development researcher with expertise in adoption, at a hearing about same-sex marriage:

> I find it offensive . . . to suggest that there's only one way of being a parent. It excludes all nonbiological parenting which would be adoptive parenting, step-parenting, foster parenting, and parenting by gay men and lesbians. . . . There are going to be some unique issues in varying forms of family. But to talk about one form of family that is best . . . is . . . offensive and a distortion of the research literature. And that's really why I'm here, you know, to make sure that message comes across (*Baehr v. Miike,* 1996, p. 31).

I find the seriousness with which Judge Chang regarded such testimony to be the most crucial aspect of his decision. In other respects, the pragmatic value of the decision is highly questionable. It comes at a time when many, including lesbians and gay men, debate the question of whether buying into the institution of legally sanctioned marriage is a progressive or regressive move. Furthermore, its power is quite limited. Currently there are 16 states that prohibit the recognition of same-sex marriages and the recently passed Defense of Marriage Act enjoins the federal government from recognizing such unions. These laws will affect gay and lesbian couples who marry in Hawaii much the same way that antimiscegenation laws affected interracial couples in the 1960s: A couple that marries in Hawaii and embarks on a cross-country trip will find themselves to be alternately married and unmarried as they cross state borders, or as *Time* magazine put it, "Some travelers will have to reset their marital status like their watches" (Kunen, 1996, p. 45). The absurdity of such a journey is an apt metaphor for the position lesbian and gay families find themselves in the landscape of the United States as we approach the millenium. Both American attitudes and law run the gamut from support to denigration, and, more often than one might imagine, these two poles coexist in the same community, even in the same psyche.

The tension between these two poles forms the context within which all families headed by lesbians or gay men currently exist. Gay men and lesbians form families under the shadow of homophobia and the idealization of the legally sanctioned, heterosexual, procreative union. At the same time, they challenge that idealization, on both profoundly private and broad public levels. The past three decades have been a time of remarkable turmoil and change with respect to the position of gay men and lesbians and the question of what constitutes a family. It is in this context of change that the experiences of gay or lesbian parents and their children must be understood.

The state's arguments in the Hawaii case were certainly not new.

They harken back to countless public denigrations of gay men and lesbians, all hinging on images of homosexuals being opposed to family life and a threat to children. In fact these two images form the basic foundation of homophobia. Thus in 1977 Anita Bryant campaigned to overturn a Dade County, Florida, ban on discrimination against homosexuals with the slogan, "Save Our Children." She called gay men and lesbians "human garbage" and criticized the civil rights ordinance as an attempt to "legitimize homosexuals and their recruitment of our children" (Matthews, Fuller, & Camp, 1977, p. 20). Her campaign resulted in repeal of the ordinance, and the very next day laws barring lesbians and gay men from marrying and adopting children were enacted ("More Cities Face Battles," 1978). Meanwhile, in California, Senator John Briggs formed the California Defend Our Children Committee, which aimed to ban gay teachers from public schools throughout the state. His rhetoric included the following: "You can act right now to help protect your family from vicious killers and defend your children from homosexual teachers. . . . Homosexuals want your children. . . . They don't have any children of their own. If they don't recruit children or very young people they'd all die away." The Briggs Initiative was defeated as a result of massive organizing efforts (Shilts, 1982, pp. 238–241).

In 1985 in Massachusetts a heated debate about lesbian and gay parenting was touched off by the removal of two foster children from the home of an openly gay couple. Though the men had been honest about their situation on their application and had been accepted by the state on those terms, once the placement of the children became public knowledge through a *Boston Globe* article (Cooper, 1985b) the children were immediately removed despite their biological mother's approval of the home. Governor Dukakis then formed a committee to review the state's policy on homosexuals as foster parents. The state developed a policy that placed "nontraditional" families at the bottom of a hierarchy and required all applicants to declare their sexual orientation. The policy clearly placed a higher value on structural as opposed to qualitative issues insofar as it favored married heterosexuals with no parenting experience over others with parenting experience (Cooper, 1985a). Despite the protests of many human service professionals who believed that foster children would suffer as a result of a policy emphasizing family structure over the quality of nurturing relationships, the policy remained in effect until 1990 (Benkov, 1994). In 1987 New Hampshire followed the examples set by Massachusetts and

Florida and enacted a law prohibiting gay men and lesbians from adopting children, becoming foster parents, or operating daycare centers. Upon passage of the bill, New Hampshire State Representative Mildred Ingram said of homosexuals, "They can go on their merry way to hell if they want to. I just want them to keep their filthy paws off the children" (Milne, 1987).

Over the years, courts in every state of the union have debated the parental fitness of homosexuals in gay and lesbian custody cases, with similar rhetoric popping up repeatedly. When lesbian custody cases first became prevalent in the 1970s, lesbians lost overwhelmingly due to one of two legal approaches: the *per se standard* held that homosexuality in and of itself was by definition reason enough to deny custody, while the *presumption of harm standard* assumed that being raised by a homosexual was damaging to children. Legal advocates pushed hard for the more fair *detriment standard,* which posits that in order for a lesbian or gay man to be denied custody due to homosexuality there must be proof that the parent's sexual orientation is harmful to the child. Though this standard has come to be more widely used, presumption of harm and per se modes of proceeding still have a strong hold in many states (Basile, 1974; Benkov, 1994; Hitchens & Price, 1978–1979; Hunter & Polikoff, 1976; Riley, 1975; Sheppard, 1985). Thus in Virginia in 1993 Sharon Bottoms lost custody of her child to her own mother solely on the grounds that her lesbianism rendered her an unfit parent in the eyes of the law.

Dramatic and violent assertions such as Anita Bryant's portrayal of homosexuals as "human garbage" represent one end of the spectrum of homophobia in American culture. Far more common, and often as harmful to gay men and lesbians, are the subtler forms of homophobia, such as the idea that it's fine to be homosexual as long as you stay in the closet, or the belief that although lesbians and gay men shouldn't be discriminated against in housing or employment, they should not be allowed to adopt children. For many, this pervasive homophobia is an obstacle to creating and maintaining familial relationships at all. For others, it constitutes, at the very least, the backdrop against which gay and lesbian parents and their children shape their families.Thus gay and lesbian parents along with their children are challenged to resist both homophobia and the idealization of the heterosexual, procreative, legally sanctioned family unit. In meeting that challenge creatively, they point toward myriad new possibilities for conceptualizing human relationships and often along the way illuminate the strength of the human spirit itself.

In reflecting on my own as well as others' experiences I have settled on four basic parameters within which one can recognize the challenges lesbian and gay parents both face and pose in the context of a culture that idealizes legally sanctioned, heterosexual, procreative unions. These parameters include the roles of gender, biology, the state, and homophobia in family life. Not all families headed by lesbians or gay men run up against dominant cultural values in each of these categories. There is diversity within the group itself, a fact that is often overlooked in discussions of these issues. For example, although many lesbians do raise children conceived through anonymous donor insemination or adoption without close male connections, thus having to contend with dominant cultural beliefs about "father absence," many other lesbian-headed families include extremely involved fathers. In the following discussion I have chosen to speak about the types of family configurations that most vividly embody the issues within each given category, but I hope the reader will nonetheless keep in mind the tremendous diversity of lesbian and gay families.

## THE ROLE OF GENDER IN FAMILY LIFE

A few years back I listened to a nationally broadcast radio talk show on single mothers by choice. In addition to a woman who had decided to raise children on her own, the guests included a psychologist who viewed women's choices to parent outside of marriage as supremely selfish acts that were clearly detrimental to children, and a man in his early 20s who had been adopted and raised by a single mother. The young man described his childhood in warm, glowing terms, having had a strong, good relationship with his mother. He noted that he had not grown up thinking about the fact that he didn't have a father or feeling attuned to what was absent from his family, but had focused instead on what was present, feeling that the only family situation he knew was indeed a good one. About midway through the broadcast the host asked the young man, "How will you know how to be a father, since you never had one yourself?" Despite having spent the first half hour eloquently describing the lessons about parent–child relationships he'd learned from his mother, the young man was stumped by the question. It didn't occur to him, or to anyone else on the program, that he had probably been well prepared for fatherhood by his mother, or, to put it another way, that he'd learned vital lessons about being a good parent through being nurtured by one. The program's participants, like many in this culture, were so riveted to the notion that parenting is fundamentally a gendered activity that they failed to recognize how much the most crucial aspects of good parenting transcend gender altogether. Can a boy learn to be a good father by experiencing and observing his mother? The answer depends greatly on what we mean by "good father" and, likewise, on what we think mothers do. The more rigidly we conceptualize parenting roles as differentially defined by gender the more likely we will be to answer "no."

This radio interchange is a prime example of the ways we as a culture overfocus on gender when we think about familial relationships, consigning both parents and children to unnecessarily limited positions. We talk about what mothers and fathers do, largely as though they are, by definition, worlds apart. And likewise, we often conceptualize the needs of boys and girls differently and focus on that difference, allowing our notions about gender to overshadow our ability to attend more fully to the needs of children both broadly and individually.

Insofar as they are socialized into gendered identities and roles in the same cultural context as others, lesbians and gay men are no less susceptible to an overfocus on limiting notions of how gender is interwoven through the fabric of family life. This is reflected in the fact that gay and lesbian family formation has mimicked the broader social pattern in which women are more likely than men to have primary parenting roles. The courts are filled with far more lesbian custody cases than those involving gay men, who are more likely to be involved in visitation disputes. Likewise, the lesbian and gay parenting boom was largely led by women, and lesbians choosing motherhood continue to far outnumber gay men choosing fatherhood.

However, at the same time as they are steeped in dominant cultural constructions of gender, over the course of their development gay men and lesbians are more likely than their heterosexual counterparts to run up against and actively resist some aspects of confining gender role definitions. This certainly can set the stage for a more complex approach to integrating gender into family life.

Both the constrictions imposed by traditional ideas about gender and the transformative power of moving beyond those ideas are vividly evident in families headed by gay men and lesbians. For example, many gay men who want children have a particularly difficult time envisioning the realization of their dream, in large part because of an internalized notion that men simply do not make good primary caretakers, particularly of very young children. There is often a process of reflection about and resistance to gendered stereotypes that accompanies gay and lesbian family formation. When gay men and lesbians raise children they are likely to run smack into the contradictions between their own deeply internalized gendered notions about parenting and new familial contexts that defy and push beyond such limited notions. This territory between two worlds can be fertile ground for fruitful examination of our assumptions about the role of gender in family life. For example, the gay father of a 2-year-old girl described his journey toward parenthood as having been sparked by an acute awareness that he'd always wanted to "be a mommy . . . to have the life [his] mother had had," a life steeped in the world of relationships and nurturance. He associated "being a mommy" particularly to the physical intimacy of caring for an infant, noting that as his daughter got older and more independent he felt increasingly more like a daddy. This was a man who had reflected a great deal on his overall values and the role of gender in his life. He felt that being gay was intricately connected to his ability to move beyond concepts of gender that limited his humanity. It is no accident that his language about the love he felt for his daughter was so steeped in gender stereotypes even as he moved beyond them.

Whereas gay men who wish to be fathers may become bogged down by the dominant notion that women, rather than men, should be primary caretakers of young children, lesbians, like unmarried heterosexual women, often mother under the burden of tremendously negative ideas about the effects of "father absence" (Polikoff, 1996). I was confronted with this early in my daughter's life, when she was just 2 days old. With my breasts rapidly swelling to twice their normal size, I headed straight from the hospital to the nearest maternity store to purchase a much-needed nursing bra. Elizabeth was in tow, along with my sister and niece. While I tried on the bra, the saleslady, pointing to Elizabeth, commented to my sister, "Shouldn't her dad be doing this?" "She doesn't have one," my sister replied. The woman appeared stricken and stumbled over the words "I'm sorry." My sister jauntily responded, "Don't be—she planned it that way." Although I had known that other people's ideas about family structure and the ways mine deviated from a norm would be something Elizabeth and I would both have to contend with, I was stunned to be faced with it so soon, while I was still basking in the extraordinary miracle of birth. The incident made me know that despite years of thinking about these issues, I had a long way to go in becoming able to respond comfortably to such encounters, particularly in a way that would provide a model for Elizabeth of how one stays proud and centered in the face of off-kilter assumptions.

The rhetoric of father absence—which holds that it reflects the breakdown of the family, is inevitably harmful to children, and is responsible for a myriad of societal ills—it is even more pointed when it comes to women raising sons. Thus perhaps the thorniest gender-related issue for lesbian parents has not only to do with gendered parenting roles but also with an overfocus on the ways gender supposedly defines children's need. The view that "father absence" is tremendously detrimental to children is held more vehemently with respect to boy children, who, it is assumed, especially need fathers to help them achieve positive male identities. Not only do many in the world around lesbian parents harbor such views, but lesbians themselves may be very vulnerable to worry about their capacity to raise healthy male children.

With the backdrop of father absence rhetoric, it is often enormously difficult for anyone to imagine that happy well-adjusted boys, comfortable in their male identities, can be raised solely by women. I was struck by this when teaching a class on lesbian and gay parents to graduate students and clinicians. I invited some children to spend an evening discussing their lives with my students. Among them was Mark, a very charming and articulate 12-year-old boy who had been conceived through anonymous donor insemination and raised from birth by his biological mother and her partner, who had recently officially adopted him. When asked if he ever felt anything was different about his family life in comparison to peers, he did not focus initially on sexual orientation but commented instead that due to the prevalence of divorce, he was one of very few children in his class being raised by the same parenting configuration he had been born into. He spoke openly about his conception through donor insemination and said that he didn't give much thought to the whole matter of fathers, commenting, "This is the only family I've known—to me it's just ordinary." Mostly he talked about his life, which included a warm immediate and extended family network, good friendships, and many interests. From all angles he was a winning child, one anybody would feel blessed to have as a son. One student, herself a lesbian mother of a young boy conceived through anonymous donor insemination, was particularly moved by the experience of listening to this child. She said it gave her hope and helped her reevaluate the guilt she felt for having brought a boy into the world who would not have a father.

On both a personal level and a larger societal one, it is hard for us to deeply question our assumptions about gender in family life. Thus we hold as a given the idea that boy children need fathers and hear much about studies purporting to demonstrate the destructive outcomes of father absence. These studies usually collapse many variables (the effects of racism, poverty, lack of education and employment opportunities, drug cultures, to name just a few) under the heading of "father absence." We hear far less about studies that show otherwise, though they do indeed exist. A Biola University study demonstrated that positive gender identity and overall outlook were not affected at all by father absence (Engber & Klungness, 1995, p. 8). Shere Hite reports anecdotally that, overall, men raised by single mothers have more positive adult relationships to women (Hite, 1995, pp. 373–374). This kind of work exists in the shadows and is given short shrift in public discourse. Lesbians parent under the burden of the societal blindness this reflects, but in raising children like Mark, they also challenge father absence rhetoric at its core.

Beyond the burdens that derive from notions about what happens when a particular gendered parenting role is "missing" from a family, lesbian and gay parents must also push beyond narrow gender-defined constructions of their own parenting roles. Although lesbians may have less difficulty than gay men recognizing and bringing to fruition their wish to be parents, they have other aspects of stereotypical gendered parenting roles to contend with. For instance, many lesbian couples raising children may struggle over how to share parenting responsibilities. This is not just a matter of logistics but rather encompasses each woman's sense of legitimacy as a mother. Often women in these situations discover that the very family they have consciously created contradicts their own deeply held view of mothers as singular, all powerful, and all important to a child. How does one share a role thus defined? Can a woman feel she is indeed a mother when she is parenting a child alongside another woman? As couples stretch themselves beyond traditional stereotypes and create arrangements that do indeed establish their family as a household headed by two mothers, they expand the very definition of motherhood itself. Likewise when gay men figure out how to run a household and raise children without wives or mothers to fall back on, they push beyond limited definitions of masculinity. These reworkings of gender-defined roles are of far-reaching significance, particularly in this time when the vast majority of heterosexual couples also need to find ways of constructing family life that do not rely on old gender definitions (Barnett & Rivers, 1996). A recent *Boston Globe* article (Meltz, 1997) reported that dual-career heterosexual couples raising children fared best in their marriage and family lives when they let go of stereotypical gender-role expectations and worked together in partnership, allowing each parent to develop and utilize skills more traditionally defined as outside their gender roles. Thus heterosexuals have a good deal to learn from lesbian and gay parenting arrangements insofar as these arrangements blatantly and creatively challenge assumptions about the inevitability of traditionally defined gender roles.

## THE ROLE OF BIOLOGICAL CONNECTION IN FAMILY LIFE

Rigidly proscribed gender roles are part and parcel not only of the idea that heterosexuality is preferable but, more specifically, of the idea that heterosexual procreation quintessentially defines family. Due to the prevalence of reproductive technologies, adoption, and families blended through divorce and remarriage, many children are raised by non-biological parents and may be in sibling relationships that are also not genetically connected. Nonetheless, families created through heterosexual procreative unions and stably maintained over time remain the central model for family, the one from which all others deviate, the standard by which all others are measured.

The story of heterosexual procreative unions is a singular one that maintains a stronghold on our psyches even as reality diverges greatly. So strong is the value we place on this model that when families come to exist in other ways we work hard to make them appear as though they result from heterosexual procreation—as though biological connections between parents and children and siblings exist. This is clear in the history of adoption practices, which until quite recently allowed access only to married couples and predominantly centered on matching physical characteristics of children to adoptive families. These practices have long been accompanied by the maintenance of secrecy about adoption itself, as though the appearance of a biologically connected unit was more important in family life than honesty. While adoption, by necessity, has evolved to include unmarried parents, cross-racial matches, and a relatively newly emerging perspective that telling the true story of adoption, with pride, is best all around, it still exists in and reflects a social context that reveres, almost fetishistically, genetic connection. The fact that many consider adoption a second-best alternative is one example of this. So too is the prevalance of stories focusing on adoptees' experiences of "missing pieces," an experience that is far from inevitable.

I once encountered a heterosexual, married woman who had three grown adopted children. She spoke with some irony about the fact that she was constantly urging her children to search for their biological parents, offering all sorts of support and help, but each would have none of it. Instead, they tried to get her to see that from their perspective she, her husband, and their siblings were all the family they wanted and needed. We do not often hear stories like this, not because they are necessarily so rare, but rather because they are given short shrift in the public discourse of a culture that idealizes genetic connection.

Donor insemination, like adoption, exists in and reflects a cultural context that overvalues the model of families formed through heterosexual procreation. In its earliest forms in this country, one of the criteria for access that many doctors utilized was an evaluation of the couple (heterosexual and married of course) with respect to their ability to keep a secret. As it is practiced today, many doctors continue to counsel that parents not tell others, including their children (Kritchevsky, 1981). Furthermore, as with older adoption practices, most often donor insemination involves careful matching of physical characteristics between donors and fathers (Noble, 1987).

Lesbian and gay parents run up against the overemphasis on biological connection in several respects. First, like all others who raise children in families that are not created through the parents' heterosexual procreation, they must contend with the idea that this is problematic. Will their children feel less than whole, as if a part of them is missing, as the story of adoptees' searches purports? Unlike many others who become parents through adoption, surrogacy, donor insemination, or remarriage, gay and lesbian parents obviously and blatantly do not fit the heterosexual procreative model. That is to say there is no possibility of the appearance of a more traditional arrangement.

It is no wonder that unmarried women, heterosexual or lesbian, had no access to donor insemination prior to the 1980s and continue to have restricted access now. Not only do prejudices about the suitability of unmarried women for motherhood play a role in this, but also the fact that when such women conceive through anonymous donor insemination there is no man to stand in as a "pretend" biological father. This is precisely the situation that was created when, due to the feminist reproductive rights movement, lesbians and other unmarried women gained access to donor insemination. When lesbians have children in this way, they must find ways to speak the truth—to their children and to the world. It is not such an easy task. One speaks into a void, a silence surrounding a practice that is over a century old, but still shrouded in secrecy. Furthermore one speaks against the backdrop of the shameful aura that surrounds donor insemination, an aura that stems from the idealization of heterosexual procreation. Perhaps most threatening is the revelation that women can conceive, bear, and raise children, with no male participation except the single contribution of sperm (Benkov, 1994).

When one finds the words to tell that story, both within and beyond the boundaries of family life, new horizons open, and so too do confrontations. This was vividly brought home to me by the daughter of some close friends. Six-year-old Julie was jumping rope with her friends in the schoolyard at recess when they struck up a conversation about their newfound knowledge of where babies come from. Someone told the 6-year-old version of heterosexual sex, conception, and birth. Julie, whose infant sister had been conceived, as she herself had, through anonymous donor insemination, piped up that the story was only one way and she knew another. She then carefully explained the process of insemination. At first her friends were disbelieving, but rather quickly they took in the information and resumed jumping rope. The next day Julie's lesbian parents got called in for a conference with the teacher. Prefacing her comments with a statement of how supportive she felt of Julie's family and of Julie herself, the teacher went on to say that she felt Julie needed to learn where she should and should not talk about these sorts of issues. The interchange was all the more striking for the fact that it occurred in an extremely liberal community and school that were known for their support of alternative family structures. Julie's parents were surprised and responded strongly. They told the teacher that in no way would they ever encourage Julie to feel or behave as though the way she had come to be on the earth were a shameful thing, not to be talked about, and they asked that the teacher take the opportunity to reflect on her own issues and remarks. This is an example of the kinds of resistance lesbian-headed families must often engage in.

Just as lesbian and gay parents who push the envelope of constricting gender roles must grapple with the contradictions between their own internalized traditional notions and the new family forms they are creating, those who confront the dominant discourse emphasizing biological connections may discover they are not only in conflict with their environment but also with themselves. Families do not always readily or easily challenge dominant notions, but instead must struggle on deeply personal levels with their own values as well as with the values of the people, communities, and institutions that surround them.

I became particularly intrigued by this when, in the process of researching my book *Reinventing the Family: The Emerging Story of Lesbian and Gay Parents* (Benkov, 1994), I encountered a wide range of approaches among lesbian couples to the question of what meaning biological connection and the lack thereof had in their families. Many defined parenting roles along biological lines, with the woman who gave birth having the status of mother while her partner was more of a friend or "aunt." Some women were content with these arrangements while others, though they created them, longed for more symmetrical role definitions. Likewise many couples defined themselves as two mothers sharing parenting responsibilities without regard to biological relationships. This group also divided into roughly two categories: those who had to work very hard to achieve this status, finding that biological connection reared its head despite their best efforts to transcend it; and those whose families, with seemingly little effort, truly did not ascribe any significance to biology.

The ways women position themselves vis-à-vis biology often constitute very active resistance to dominant discourse. This is evident in families that consciously try to balance the physical connection engendered by nursing by having the other mother be physically close through bath giving; or families that carefully educate their neighbors to inquire of their children, "How are your mommies?" rather than "How is your mommy?"; or families that decide not to honor questions such as, "Who is the biological mom?" with an answer other than "We're both moms." Likewise, many children from such families carry on their own resistance. To peers who asked her which was her real mother, one 9-year-old girl described responding that both were her real mothers because "a mother is the person who loves and takes care of you, not just the person who gave birth." What gay and lesbian families thus demonstrate so vividly then is that biology itself is not nearly so important as what we make of it, and what we make of it is a social creation, not an individual one (Benkov, 1994).

## THE ROLE OF THE STATE IN FAMILY LIFE

Families grow out of the possibilities inherent in their contexts, but as people struggle mightily to transform themselves and go against the grain of dominant ideas, they bring their private transformations into the world. These come in the form of living, breathing children with their own consciousness, and in the form of public discourse, reflected through changes in media, school curriculum, medical practices, and law.

The fact that families are not self-defined in a vacuum is abundantly clear when one looks at lesbian and gay situations. The power of the state to shape family life is often formidable. Law determines custody in cases of death or divorce and plays a role in who has access to adoption and reproductive technologies. Furthermore the question of whether families that exist are recognized as such is of major pragmatic and philosophical importance. Children of gay and lesbian parents are rendered extremely vulnerable by the lack of legal recognition granted to the families' primary relationships. Insofar as the law relies heavily on the idealization of the legally sanctioned, heterosexual, procreative union, the relationships that are most often recognized by the state are biological, or formed in the context of heterosexual marriage. When lesbian or gay couples split up, their children are highly likely to be seen as having only one parent, the biological or legally adoptive one. Likewise, nonbiological sibling relationships go unrecognized. This has left many children facing traumatic losses. Similarly, when a biological or legally adoptive parent dies, children may be put in the care of relatives to whom they have little relation rather than in the care of their remaining parent, who lacks legal status (Polikoff, 1990).

There are two aspects of resistance that emerge in the face of the discontinuities between families' self-definitions and the state. The first is a challenge to lesbian and gay parents, one they may meet or fall far short of. It requires a heightened sense that the core of family values lies in something no one can legislate. It lies in trust and commitment among family members regardless of how others define their relationships. Thus many couples articulate the knowledge that it will be up to them to honor each other's connections to children in the event of a split because the law is not likely to do so. Of course many families do not live according to such principles, especially in moments of crisis, and that is one reason that change in the public domain is so critical to children's well-being. The other reason is that children are vulnerable to extended family members and communities who do not recognize their most crucial relationships.

The second mode of resistance to conflicting definitions of family is the fight for legal recognition of diverse family forms. Since the mid-1980s, lesbians and gay men have made strides with respect to the use of "second-parent adoptions," whereby both couple members can have legally recognized parental status (Bashaw, 1990; Patt, 1988; Zuckerman, 1986). Furthermore, though it is not yet common, courts are more frequently recognizing "psychological parents" as people with rights to custody or visitation in the case of death or splits (Polikoff, 1990). These kinds of changes are not only tremendously important to children raised by lesbians and gay men, but also have broader significance. Gay and lesbian parents are among the many people whose "nontraditional" families are leading the state itself to have to reconsider the fundamental question of what constitutes a family. Increasingly, particular configurations of gender and biology are giving way to more qualitative criteria. Thus very private struggles are sparking transformation of the larger culture.

## THE ROLE OF HOMOPHOBIA IN FAMILY LIFE

For several years preceding the birth of my daughter, I had occasion to pore over newspaper clippings, law articles, psychological studies, and court transcripts involving lesbian and gay parents. Many included rhetoric essentially describing me and some of my closest friends in monstrous terms. Though I experienced a kind of moral outrage, for the most part I read these descriptions calmly and nonchalantly. Was it familiarity that led to this demeanor, the boredom that comes with endless repetition? It was not until I read the Hawaii decision that I turned to reflect on the discrepancy between my cool response and the disturbing nature of the rhetoric and its effects. Familiarity was only part of the story.

There is such a vast distance between cardboard villifications and the complexity of lesbian and gay lives that it is difficult to make the association to one's own life when faced with such rhetoric. Therein lies the great chasm that prejudice of any kind creates between lives known from the inside deeply and fully, and lives described from the outside through a filter of ignorance. This accounts for some, but not all, of my emotional distance. It is also important that I have been very fortunate not to have my family life dramatically affected by the most vehement forms of homophobia—I have never been denied the possibility of conception or adoption, faced a custody loss threat, or felt myself or my children to be physically unsafe. Although this plays a crucial role in my cool demeanor, there is yet another dimension that warrants exploration. In a way, remaining calm and oddly untouched by such violent distortion of one's own life is, in and of itself, a form of resistance. Like the child we, as parents, hope to learn to walk away from a schoolyard bully, I choose many times to walk away emotionally from denigration born of ignorance, fear, and hatred. I choose to do so in order to focus my energies on the people, activities, and ideas I love—in other words to live my life as I define it, not in reaction to bigotry.

When Elizabeth was just beginning to learn how to talk she was entranced by a tape of Danny Kaye singing *The Ugly Duckling,* insisting it be played over and over. One of her very first sentences, in exact imitation of the delighted voice with which he said this, was "Yes, I *am* a swan." For a while it was like a mantra, repeated after every question to which there was an affirmative answer: "Elizabeth, do you want ice cream?" "Yes," pause, "I *am* a swan." She got me to thinking. The story of the ugly duckling is essentially a story of prejudice; a swan judged in a duck context is deemed "ugly." Internalizing the taunts of others it becomes sad and isolated. Freed from the defining context and discovering others like itself, it emerges joyously recognizing its own true nature and beauty. Elizabeth is my swan. I want for her always to know that every aspect of her is, in its own way, sacred. It is something many parents in this culture want for their children: that they feel good about themselves, both valued and valuable. For lesbian and gay parents, as for all others who deviate in some way that is negatively valued in a dominant context, this wish is poignant and not so easy to achieve.

Gay and lesbian parents have often traversed their own difficult path toward self-acceptance and pride. How do they help their children do the same? Through conversation they build the foundation for understanding that prejudice exists and that it is a problem, rather than the objects of discrimination being the problem. Those who can also try early on to control environments as much as possible, situating their children in contexts that reflect and honor diversity, and helping them know other similarly structured families. Many don't have the luxury of doing this by virtue of being geographically isolated, under threat of custody or job loss, without family support, or economically limited in their choices.

No matter what kinds of environments parents carefully create for their young children, as children age, they make their own connections and interact in wider and wider circles of society. They may go through their own homophobic periods, requiring parents to think not only about protecting them from prejudice but also about children as the potential vehicle through which homophobia enters the heart of family life. This can be very thorny, particularly when combined with adolescent concerns about peer acceptance and separation from family. When a child asks parents to refrain from holding hands around his friends, how much do parents play along, how much do they resist in order to honor their own values, modeling pride and zero tolerance of homophobia? As parents and children traverse this difficult territory the stage is set for crucial life lessons. The ways families confront homophobia can provide the foundation for children to achieve the capacity to think independently, to develop compassion, to recognize the connections among marginalized groups, and to understand the value and power of resistance.

## THE CHALLENGES LESBIAN AND GAY PARENTS POSE

I believe lesbian and gay parents challenge society not only with respect to the four domains described above but also with respect to a deeper set of issues. By their very existence, these families make the point that the quality of our interactions matters far more than conformity to any particular structure, that difference is valuable rather than problematic, that lives are complex and can't be simply categorized, and that it is worth getting to know people rather than blindly accepting myths about them.

Elizabeth has entered the stage of endless questions, a newfound pleasure she particularly likes to engage in at bedtime. One night she came padding out of her room with the 14th question of the evening: "Mommy, someday will you be a language instead of a mommy?" Anxious to get her back to bed, I answered hastily, "No, Elizabeth, I'll always be your mommy." But as usual no sooner had she drifted off to sleep than I began to reflect on her seemingly nonsensical query. All of a sudden it made perfect sense, and I felt I'd answered incompletely. Suddenly I saw a time when the moments we now share together would be in her memory rather than her present. With that image in mind I realized that, of course, I hope someday to be a language for her, or more aptly, that we together will be a language—one she knows deeply in her soul, one she takes pride in, one she can add to or change, one she can teach others. I hope it is a language of vision, joy, love, and strength.

## REFERENCES

Baehr v. Miike, No. 91-1394 (Hi. Cir. Ct. 1996) (WL694 235).

Barnett, R., & Rivers, C. (1996). *She works, he works: How two-income families are happier, healthier, and better off.* New York: HarperCollins.

Bashaw, C. (1990). Protecting children in nontraditional families: Second parent adoptions in Washington. *University of Puget Sound Law Review, 13*, 321–347.

Basile, R. A. (1974). Lesbian mothers I. *Women's Rights Law Reporter, 2*, 3–18.

Benkov, L. (1994). *Reinventing the family: The emerging story of lesbian and gay parents.* New York: Crown.

Cooper, K. (1985a, May 25). New policy on foster care. *The Boston Globe*, p. 1.

Cooper, K. (1985b, May 8). Some oppose foster placement with gay couple. *The Boston Globe*, p. 21.

Engber, A., & Klungness, L. (1995). *The complete single mother.* Holbrook, MA: Adams Media.

Hitchens, D., & Price, B. (1978–1979). Trial strategy in lesbian mother custody cases: The use of expert testimony. *Golden Gate University Law Review, 9*, 451–479.

Hite, S. (1995). *The Hite report on the family: Growing up under patriarchy.* New York: Grove/Atlantic.

Hoeffer, B. (1981). Children's acquisition of sex role behavior in lesbian mother families. *American Journal of Orthospsychiatry, 51*(3), 536–544.

Hunter, N., & Polikoff, N. (1976). Custody rights of lesbian mothers: Legal theory and litigation strategy. *Buffalo Law Review, 25*, 691–733.

Kirkpatrick, M., Smith, C., & Roy, R. (1981). Lesbian mothers and their children: A comparative survey. *American Journal of Orthopsychiatry, 51*(3), 545–551.

Kritchevsky, B. (1981). The unmarried woman's right to artificial insemination: A call for an expanded definition. *Harvard Women's Law Journal, 4*, 1–22.

Kunen, J. (1996, December 16). Hawaiian courtship. *Time*, pp. 44–45.

Kweskin, S., & Cook, A. (1982). Heterosexual and homosexual mothers' self-described sex role behavior and ideal sex role behavior in children. *Sex Roles, 8*(9), 967–975.

Matthews, T., Fuller, T., & Camp, H. (1977, June 6). Battle over gay rights. *Newsweek*, p. 20.

Meltz, B. (1997, January 2). The delicate balance of two-income families. *The Boston Globe*, p. D12.

Miller, J., Jacobsen, B., & Bigner, J. (1981). The child's home environment for lesbian versus heterosexual mothers: A neglected area of research. *Journal of Homosexuality, 7*(1), 49–56.

Milne, J. (1987, July 24). Starting today New Hampshire bars gay foster parents. *The Boston Globe*, p. 13.

More cities face battles over homosexual rights. (1978, May 28). *The New York Times,* p. 36.

Noble, E. (1987). *Having your baby by donor insemination: A complete resource guide.* Boston: Houghton Mifflin.

Pagelow, M. (1980). Heterosexual and lesbian single mothers: A comparison of problems, coping and solutions. *Journal of Homosexuality, 5*(3), 551–572.

Patt, E. (1987). Second parent adoption: When crossing the marital barrier is in a child's best interests. *Berkeley Women's Law Journal, 3,* 96–133.

Patterson, C. (1992). Children of lesbian and gay parents. *Child Development, 63*(5), 1025–1042.

Polikoff, N. (1990). This child does have two mothers: Redefining parenthood to meet the needs of children in lesbian-mother and other nontraditional families. *Georgetown Law Journal, 78,* 459–575.

Polikoff, N. (1996). The deliberate construction of families without fathers: Is it an option for lesbian and heterosexual mothers? *Santa Clara Law Review, 36*(2), 375–394.

Rand, C., Graham, D., & Rawlings, E. (1982). Psychological health and factors the court seeks to control in lesbian mother custody trials. *Journal of Homosexuality, 8*(1), 27–39.

Riley, M. (1975). The avowed lesbian and her right to child custody: A challenge that can no longer be denied. *San Diego Law Review, 12,* 806–857.

Sheppard, A. T. (1985). Lesbian mothers II: Long night's journey into day. *Women's Rights Law Reporter, 8*(4), 218–246.

Shilts, R. (1982). *The mayor of Castro Street: The life and times of Harvey Milk.* New York: St. Martin's Press.

Zuckerman, E. (1986). Second parent adoption for lesbian-parented families: Legal recognition of the other mother. *University of California Davis Law Review, 19*(3), 729–759.

# 6

## Safeguarding Wordless Voice in a World of Words

*BONNIE Y. OHYE*

*I AM* a dark-haired, dark-eyed woman of Japanese ancestry. I married a blonde, blue-eyed man of Anglo-European ancestry whose paternal ancestors arrived in America in the 1600s. By training, I am a child psychologist, and by good fortune, I am the mother of two daughters, one 9 and one 2 years old. It has been an important epiphany as a mother to recognize that in spite of being two generations removed from my grandparents' journeys from Japan, I am nonetheless living an immigrant's tale. As such, it is a tale of assimilation and accommodation, a story of being "on both shores at once" (Anzaldua, 1987, p. 78). Straddling this shifting and intricate landscape means holding contradictory impulses—to embrace what is different, yet not relinquish oneself in that openness; to preserve, yet to welcome transformation. I draw on the memories of my grandmothers and mother, who, within the context of their respective generations in America, found ways to nurture, protect, and prepare their children to travel back and forth across the cultural border.

My understanding of my struggle to achieve this valuing of two cultures with my own children has been slowly and painfully achieved. The writing of this chapter represents a unique moment in my own history, a place where I can give credence to an individual story as opposed to the accumulated weight of many other individual stories. It is a struggle that is intimately related to the bidding of my Japanese heritage to dissolve one's "self" in order to uphold the communal order. Coming to this place has entailed bearing the murmured prohibitions of my heritage against drawing attention to oneself. I do so now in order to articulate a question that has become increasingly central in my thoughts as a mother. That question is "Will my children hear my 'voice' if I do not speak?"

How difficult it has been to learn to lean on words! Japanese children are reminded by their mothers, *Mono ieba kuchibiru samushi aki no kaze* (If you talk, your lips will feel cold). It has been said that Japanese consider writing "an act of defiance against the cultural norm of silence" (Lebra, 1987). This seems, of course, to be a wild exaggeration. But why then do I feel instant recognition when I read the appreciation of a Korean American woman for mentors "who never mistook my slowness of speech for imbecility" (Cheung, 1993, p. xii)? Or, why my emotional resonance with the experience of someone learning English as a second language: "It takes all my will to impose any control on the words that emerge from me. I have to form entire sentences before uttering them; otherwise, I too easily get lost in the middle" (Hoffman, 1989, p. 118)?

I wish to suggest the possibility that a mother's "voice" can be heard without speech, that knowing another can occur in a context that does not emphasize speaking, and that my children will come to discern much about their mother and her heritage through silence. This silence is not that of a drowned or silenc*ed* voice, but rather is silence that is eloquent and resonant, embedded within a universe that steadily and powerfully directs one's attention away from the "self" to the "other."

This universe holds the ideal of knowing another through quiet observation and of being known by another without speaking. It is a universe of abiding trust in the other's capacity to satisfy one's wishes. I love the comfort and familiarity of this world and hope my children will know something of it, too. It is impossible, however, to hold myself apart from Western culture's prizing of speech, words, talking, and action. We all are expected to learn the importance of "speaking one's mind" as a skill necessary for success, verbal self-assertion as a mark of healthy self-esteem, and articulate speech as a reflection of intelligence. Yet, to claim the instructive value in my individual life is to threaten the universe in which I was raised. It is the tension between the morality of collectivity and the morality of individualism and its expressions in the life of my family that increasingly occupy my thoughts as a mother. Imparting the value to my children of both these ways of being in the world is without question the most arduous work in my mothering. It is the experience of the strain in that work that I hope to describe for you.

My thoughts about this question are deepened by the writings of social scientist mothers like Weingarten (1997; also Chapter 1, this volume) and Benkov (1994; also Chapter 5, this volume), who have directed our attention to social context as intimately related to the nature of our experiences, the judgments we bear upon them, and how we feel about ourselves. The contributions of psychologists such as Kagitçibasi (1990, 1994) and Markus and Kitayama (1991, 1994), with their concepts of the psychology of relatedness and those of the *interdependent* versus the *independent* self-construals, respectively, are sources of great intellectual comfort and guidance.

The frame of reference for the thinking and feeling that accompanies this aspect of my maternal work has been pieced together in anything but a linear fashion, drawing on conversations with other mothers, literary writings, the analytic paradigms of my training as a clinical psychologist and, more recently, those from anthropology and cultural psychology. All have informed and helped shape my thinking. I begin by placing my experience in a framework from anthropology and, specifically, in relationship to the concepts of individualism and collectivism. From these broad contrasts of the individualist and the collectivist orientations, I turn to the generational and familial context within which I became a mother. Lastly, I describe three moments in which I find myself poised between two "shores" that, for my children, I strive to hold together without diminishing, disparaging, or rejecting either.

## THE TWO SHORES: INDIVIDUALISM AND COLLECTIVISM

Hoefstede defines individualism and collectivism as follows: "Individualism pertains to societies in which the ties between individuals are loose: everyone is expected to look after himself or herself and his or her immediate family. Collectivism as its opposite pertains to societies in which people from birth onwards are integrated into strong, cohesive ingroups, which throughout people's lifetime continue to protect them in exchange for unquestioning loyalty" (1991, p. 51). Individualist cultures emphasize self-knowledge, personal responsibility, personal fulfillment, and self-reliance. Collectivist cultures, on the other hand, emphasize the individual's connection to the natural world and to other people, emotional dependence, sharing, duties, and obligations.

It is widely accepted that Japan is a collectivist culture; its cultural value system has distinctive notions that sustain its particular collective orientation. A full characterization of Japanese culture is outside the scope of this chapter. For this I would refer you to the work of eminent Japan scholars such as Benedict (1946), Doi (1973), Barnlund (1975), and Lebra (1976). I draw here instead on the impressive work of sociolinguist Wierzbicka (1991) and her colleagues in order to provide a concise glimpse into the Japanese culture.

In applying her culture-independent framework based on semantic primitives (e.g., "I," "you," "want," "think," "good," "bad"), Wierzbicka (1991) identifies six concepts essential to understanding the Japanese cultural value system. They are *amae* (trustful dependence), *enryo* (discretion, modesty, polite hesitation), *wa* (harmony within the group), *on* (obligation, favor), *giri* (the moral imperative to perform one's duties to one's group), and *seishin* (fortitude). In spite of the highly simplified nature of these linguistic windows, one senses a culture in which an individual's attention is directed outward from the self to the surrounding web of social relationships and the attendant obligations and benefits.

These values are evident when Japanese parents are asked to describe the quality they most wish to nurture in their children. They speak of *sunao,* an open-hearted cooperation through sensitivity with the other. For example, when children in Japan are being coaxed to eat their evening meal, they are likely to be urged to "think about the farmer who worked so hard to produce this rice for you; if you don't eat it, he will feel bad, for his efforts will have been in vain" (Yamada, 1986, cited in Markus & Kitayama, 1991, p. 224). Mothers in the United States are likely to assert their authority when a child is behaving inappropriately, whereas mothers in Japan invariably appeal to the child's feelings for others and to the interpersonal consequences of their actions, for example, "If you make noise in the supermarket the grocer will become upset because he works hard to make the market a nice place to shop."

By early childhood, Japanese children identify interpersonal responsibility as the most important quality in a "good" child (Kashiwagi & Azuma, 1971, cited in Yeh, 1995). When presented with Kohlberg's (1969) standard tasks of moral reasoning, Japanese adolescents offer solutions that reflect a relational orientation more often than their American counterparts (Yamagishi, 1976, cited in Yeh, 1995; Araki & Yoshida, 1985, cited in Yeh, 1995). It is important to note that this relationship-focused standard of moral correctness characteristic of collectivist cultures is not "discretionary" as it is in the United States, but is the expectation for boys as well as girls (e.g., Miller, 1994).

Several scholars, most notably, Triandis (1989), Kagitçibashi (1990, 1994), and Markus and Kitayama (1991, 1994), have made substantial contributions to the theoretically challenging task of linking the broad level of cultural description afforded by the concepts of individualism and collectivism to that of individual psychology. Markus and Kitayama have taken contrasts between Japan and the United States as their point of theoretical departure, and so their work in this area has been especially relevant and provocative to my thinking. I would like to describe briefly their ideas most pertinent to this discussion.

Markus and Kitayama (1991, 1994) suggest that self-definition or *self-construal* most parsimoniously explains the psychological differences between individuals socialized in individualistic cultures and those from collectivist cultures. They argue that when the fundamental cultural goal is for individuals to function autonomously, then one is required to make behavior, thoughts, and feelings meaningful primarily in reference to the self's own thoughts, feelings, and actions rather than in relationship to those of others. They regard this self-construal as the *independent self*. Alternatively, in collectivist cultures, the cultural goal is in-group harmony and appropriate social relationships. The meaning of individual actions, feelings, and behavior is most completely realized and most satisfactorily experienced in connection with others. This self-definition is referred to as the *interdependent self* construal.

In clarifying the contrast between these self-construals, Markus and Kitayama suggest that "it may not be unreasonable to suppose . . . that in some cultures, on certain occasions, the individual, in the sense of a set of significant inner attributes of the person, may cease to be the primary unit of consciousness. Instead, the sense of belongingness to a social relation may become so strong that it makes better sense to think of the *relationship* as the functional unit of conscious reflection" (1991, p. 226, emphasis in the original). They go on to marshal compelling empirical support for their assertion that these two self-experiences are systematically associated with differences in cognition, motivation, and emotion.

The cross-cultural developmental literature abundantly illustrates that the socialization practices in Japan support the cultural aims of fitting in harmoniously with others, being receptive to the initiatives of others, and nurturing concern for others. Japanese mothers and their children are engaged in a relationship in which interdependence is its hallmark. In their review of comparative studies of the parent–child relationship in Japan and the United States, Fogel, Stevenson, and Messinger (1994) conclude, "The degree of interdependence fostered between parent and child in Japan *cannot be underestimated*" (p. 49, emphasis in original).

This interdependence, for instance, can be discerned in studies comparing Japanese and U.S. infants' response to the Strange Situation paradigm (e.g., Miyake, Campos, Kagan, & Bradshaw, 1985). In this experimental situation, Japanese infants are found to be more likely to respond to distress by orienting to the mother, whereas distressed U.S. infants turn more consistently to the environment as reflected by behaviors such as manipulation of toys. In a comparison of mother–toddler problem-solving style, Messinger (1992) observed that American toddlers more frequently demonstrated a desire to do the task without maternal assistance or direction; Japanese mother–child pairs, by contrast, worked more consistently together as a single problem-solving unit. This closely aligned relationship between mother and child undoubtedly serves as the experiential context in which children develop their capacity for discerning the interpersonal cues that guide socially appropriate action, thus preparing them for participation in the larger culture.

Significantly, it appears that fostering the deep bond between mother and child is effected much more prominently through nonverbal means (e.g., gestures, touch, facial expression) than through verbal means (Clancy, 1986; Toda, Fogel, & Kawai, 1990). Japanese mothers, for example, "chat" less to their quiet infants than do mothers in the United States (e.g., Caudill & Weinstein, 1969). Their speech appears to have less information content but more affective content than that of U.S. mothers; when a Japanese mother does speak to her infant, she is more likely than an American mother to be greeting the child, calling the child by name, singing songs, or using onomatopoeics. She is also more likely to be using speech to encourage or discourage rather than, as is the tendency observed in mothers in the United States, to identify, report, and interpret the events and experiences in the environment for the baby. She more likely will identify and comment on the baby's state rather than aspects of the environment (e.g., Fogel et al., 1994). Finally, Japanese mothers do not rely upon verbal direction and guidance as prominently as do mothers in the United States in order to garner compliance from their children. Instead, Japanese mothers much more frequently than mothers in the United States instruct their children through example (Azuma, 1986; Fogel et al.,

1994), or as I would reframe it from the perspective of the child, through quiet observation.

Indeed, I see the legacy of "silent" Japanese mothers in this observation of my own family: My then 2-year-old, eyeing a forbidden activity, was asked by her daycare mother, "What would your mom say?" Her response was not "No-no-no." Instead, she screwed up her little face, wrinkling her nose, frowning, and scrunching her eyebrows together in imitation of the prohibition and disapproval she must see in my own face.

## OUR FAMILIES OF ORIGIN: FROM TWO SHORES

I see the power and adaptive function of the collectivist tenets in my own history. Their expression is an ethic of interpersonal relationships such as interdependence, sharing, duties, obligation, and family loyalty, which is communicated through means other than "talk." These collectivist tenets were reinforced for me by two factors. The first is the legacy of the fact that my grandparents, parents, and their siblings had been sent to internment camps during World War II. The second is the economic hardship of being raised in a mother-only household (see McLoyd, 1990). I can see that both racism and socioeconomic status contributed significantly to the collectivist imperatives in my life. However, although these might be discerned in what follows, I would like to place them in the background as I try to bring other elements to the foreground.

My four grandparents immigrated from Japan in the early 1900s. My father's parents established a farm in the Central Valley of California; my mother's parents a small strawberry farm on Bainbridge Island, Washington. My father was one of three children; my mother one of eight. In 1942, both families were "relocated" from their homes to internment camps, my maternal grandparents to Manzanar, California, and my paternal grandparents to Poston, Arizona. Following the war, my paternal grandparents reestablished themselves in Oakland, California, involving their three children in a family-run business. My maternal grandparents sought refuge, as did many from Manzanar, in a church-sponsored shelter, "the hostel" in Los Angeles, and remained in Los Angeles. I was raised in a large, highly interdependent, extended family that consisted of my grandparents, five aunts, six uncles, eight cousins, my mother, and my own younger sister and two younger brothers.

My husband's ancestry is English, Irish, and German. His father's ancestors immigrated from England in the 17th century; his paternal grandmother was a descendent of Patrick Henry. His father was a career chemical engineer and his mother, a full-time wife and mother of three, two girls and a boy. In contrast to the collectivist tenets with which I was raised, they raised their only son to be an exemplar of rugged individualism as reflected by self-sufficiency, individual achievement through competition, and emotional independence from others.

When we married, John and I were each extremely naive about the task that was ahead of us as we joined our lives and our cultural traditions. It never occurred to us that it would be difficult. After all, we were both educated in the public schools of California, went on to earn postgraduate degrees, our families were both Protestant, I spoke English, he didn't need to speak Japanese, and we grew up in California with its remarkable diversity of racial and ethnic groups. But perhaps most falsely comforting were John's "sensitivity" and my apparent ease with an individualist orientation as reflected in my academic accomplishment and "successful" separation and individuation from my family.

Here is an exchange that captures the central cultural and relational chasm that our marriage made manifest:

JOHN: If you would only have *asked* me to do that. . . . I can't be expected to "read your mind."

BONNIE: (*with bewilderment and sometimes tears*) Why is it so hard for you to know that it is important to me and do it *without my asking*?

I sought counsel and affirmation among other professional wives. Their response was one of the following: (1) It's gender. Men aren't trained to be attentive to emotional needs; they aren't taught to be nurturing; or (2) you *do* need to tell him what you want him to do.

Neither of these ways of understanding our conflict was comforting, clarifying, or helpful. When I was finally able to tell John what I had expected, he was usually responsive, attentive, and nurturing. However, the act of making my needs known through "direct verbal expression" made me feel unhappy. I felt I was being compelled to participate in our relationship in a way that did not feel natural.

In contrast to my friends' counsel, I have found comfort and clarity in the following contrasting descriptions of a brief exchange between two friends. They are discussing what the guest would like to have his American host prepare for lunch (Markus & Kitayama, 1991, p. 229).

*Conversation 1*

HOST:  Hey, Tom, what do you want in your sandwich? I have turkey, salami, and cheese.

TOM:  Oh, I like turkey.

*Conversation 2 (between host and a visitor from Japan)*

HOST:  Hey, Tomio, what do you want in your sandwich? I have turkey, salami, and cheese.

TOMIO:  (*a little moment of bewilderment and then a noncommittal utterance like*) I don't know.

*Conversation 3 (between Japanese host and Tomio)*

HOST:  Hey, Tomio, I made you a turkey sandwich because I remember you like turkey more than beef.

TOMIO:  Oh, thank you, I really like turkey.

My husband expected our negotiations to proceed as in the first conversation. I was to know what I wanted and I would state it. For many things, I did, and things proceeded smoothly. However, in those matters of greatest emotional importance, often they did not. In these matters, the matters closest to my heart, my expectation of him was that he was closely attending to my needs, anticipating what I needed, and would provide it without my asking. And, I expected no less from myself in relationship to his comforts and needs.

The novelist Kogawa (1981) writes of her experience as the recipient of such care: "The most reliable map I am given [to understand propriety of action] is the example of my mother's and Grandma's alert and accurate knowing. When I am hungry, and before I can ask, there is food. If I am weary, every place is a bed. . . . A sweater covers me before there is any chill and if there is pain there is care simultaneously" (p. 68).

And with respect to emotional needs, she writes: "All the while that she acts, there is calm efficiency in her face—the eyes of Japanese motherhood. They do not invade and betray. They are eyes that protect, shielding what is hidden most deeply in the heart of the child. She makes safe the small stirrings underfoot and in the shadows" (Kogawa, 1981, p. 71).

These passages, I believe, also reveal Kogawa's experience of the wordless fostering of the tie between child and mother and how deeply embedded that connection is within a universe that directs one to feel and think what the other is thinking and feeling, to absorb information without being told, and then to help the other satisfy their wishes. Maintaining this tie requires inhibiting the "I" perspective and giving primacy to the "thou" perspective (Hsu, 1981).

My children hold out to me the challenge of honoring the traditions of my heritage as I, along with their father, other family members, and friends, prepare them to be comfortable and skillful in their lifetime of relationships. I know my daughters are most likely to encounter the interpersonal assumptions of the individualist orientation in the contexts of their growing up: school, the workplace, church, political affiliation, and perhaps in their own lifelong partnerships. So, rightly or wrongly, I have set myself the task of making choices about my expectations and responses in my mothering in order to support interpersonal competencies that are "instrumental" in our society.

I take deeply to heart Ruddick's analysis of the challenges of rearing children in our society: "Many mothers find that the central challenge of mothering lies in training a child to be the kind of person whom others accept and whom the mothers themselves can actively appreciate" (1989, p. 104). In reading this observation, I feel fortified against the many concerns about this choice as a mother. It helps me feel less alone during the hard times of being a mother between cultures by extending to me the capacious shelter of the community of mothers across time, across place, and across circumstance. But before I can take a breath, the phrase "the kind of person . . . whom the mothers themselves can actively appreciate" intrudes on my rest. It urges me to find ways to impart to my daughters some of the notions of good and worthy action that dwell within me. The peril in not doing so is to render them unfamiliar, outside the intimacy of feeling "at home" (Weingarten, 1997) with someone you love.

I share with you now three memories in which I see myself working as a mother to hold these two aspects in equipoise, finding a way to affirm the wisdom in my cultural tradition while acknowledging the differences between the expectations that surrounded me and those that surround my children.

## "I DID THIS BECAUSE YOU ARE MY MOTHER"

Mine was a hierarchical world in which elders' decisions were rarely questioned. If you were a mother in this world, it was unnecessary to appeal to reason, unnecessary to make a clearly articulated request. It was sufficient that you were a mother. Compliance in this world feels right, it feels good. Being dutiful brings feelings of being in harmony with the moral order and closeness to others. Conroy, Hess, Azuma, and Kashiwagi (1980) observe that the child in Japanese culture is trained for compliance not through analysis or questioning, but by fostering a desire to please the mother. I recognize, however, that this kind of interaction is a continuity from my upbringing that will likely not serve my children well. Compliance to authority is more ambivalently regarded in the contexts in which my daughters will develop and grow. According to the culturally dominant standard, children are expected to learn to assert themselves directly, albeit respectfully, in relationship to authority figures, and to derive feelings of mastery and self-enhancement as the natural consequences of their skillful negotiations (Weisz, Rothbaum, & Blackburn, 1984). Knowing this, I have decided to try to use words to foster with my children expectations about how relationships are conducted within a world with individualist values.

Sometimes I despair that I will accomplish this, however, when I find the following statement utterly exhausting to think up and say: "Eliza, would you please remember to pick up the things from your bedroom floor by tomorrow morning because otherwise I won't be able to vacuum your room."

This structuring of her relationship to my expectations works because Eliza has come to believe (1) she is entitled to have an explanation for my expectations, (2) she expects that I will make a reasonable demand, and (3) she expects that I will respect her personal autonomy.

These expectations feel very strange. I did not relate to my mother's requests as something separate from her, as something that could be evaluated for their logic and degree of mutuality. My mother's requests were my mother, and thus my actions were a direct statement about my feelings for her. The notion that a mother could *love* her child, but not like her child's *behavior* did not exist in my growing up.

Thus, it is an effort to remember that the rules are different for Eliza. I work diligently to word my request completely even as I remember visits from my sister and brother during which they chide

Eliza for not immediately responding to me, "Eliza, your mother asked you to do something." I work at this even as I am wishing she would do it not because I am a reasonable mother, but because I am her mother. But perhaps my hard work is misguided, for Eliza still searches my face and asks, "Mom, are you tired? You just sighed."

## *"SO, YOU THINK I SHOULD FEEL SORRY FOR HER?"*

My 9-year-old earlier this year had a friend who sought her out at every recess, demanding that they play exclusively together. This child is also the child of neighbors, and therefore has a very significant relationship to my daughter and to our family.

In my talk with my daughter I found myself asking her what her feelings were and also encouraging her to imagine her friend's feelings. Eliza could sense that this conversation might lead to a conclusion she was not entirely happy about, one that would subordinate her feelings to those of her friend, and she blurted out, "So, you think I should feel sorry for her?! I feel sorry for myself!"

I felt trapped. I could exert my influence as her mother and answer in the way that felt congruent with my own upbringing and its emphasis upon maintaining harmony within relationships to others at all costs, and the attendant idea that pursuing harmony demonstrates maturity, tolerance, and self-control. But it was quite obvious that answering in this way would incur the loss of my daughter's confidence that I had heard her feelings. Alternatively, I could side with her feelings and let her know that she had my permission to "take care of herself" and that her friend should be held to the same individualist standard. I could sense that this is what she wanted to hear. Yet, I could not bring myself to endorse this standard with my whole heart. For doing so carried the risk of casting my child and her actions outside that which I had been trained to embrace as good, worthy, and honorable. I could not relinquish this part of me; neither could I give her over completely to the other.

Instead, we embarked on a lengthy discussion of ways to accommodate both her feelings and those of her friend. She decided that she would try to incorporate her friend into the group activities she was involved with for a while, so as to foster other friendships. If her friend's requests continued, she would say something like, "I don't mean to hurt your feelings, but today I'd like to play with 'so-and-so' instead."

This resolution helped us both. It is harder to incorporate both the collectivist ethic and the individualist ethic rather than simply to assert one or the other. When I am most honest, I can admit that I wish I could have it my own way; it would be easier on me. But my way only works if the social context supports it and espouses it, and I see, and my child lets me know, that hers is a context different from the one in which I was raised. I suppose the peace I have made about this private loss has something to do with holding the expectation that Eliza will act without malice even as she feels the freedom not to subordinate her needs in order to demonstrate her maturity and tolerance. But as I realize how much her question was in fact a declaration—"So *you* think I should feel sorry for her!"—I wonder how free to "feel sorry for herself" I can really help her to be.

## "SHE'S SO FULL OF LIFE!"

My daughter's second-grade teacher offered this as a description of my child the day after school was out for summer vacation. It was a beautiful, sunny day, and we were both in the town produce market shopping for fruit. "She's so full of life," she said with warmth and as a compliment. I reciprocated by expressing appreciation for her warmth and skill as a teacher.

Beneath my calm exterior my immediate and instinctive response was alarm. "She must be showing too much of herself," I thought. "This will only bring disaster." To stand out from the group is shameful. Fitting in harmoniously is the ideal. Maturity is expressed by *controlling* the social expression of opinions, abilities, and characteristics (Markus & Kitayama, 1991); attention to individual characteristics and accomplishments should be subordinated to the sense of group integrity and collective identity.

I recognize that the larger social context of my daughter's life would find my reactions odd, even incomprehensible. The belief in the necessity of praise, reward, and positive reinforcement and the unshakable conviction that positive self-esteem is to be cultivated are so deeply positioned in our culture that it is evident even in the earliest interactions between parents and their infants (Brazelton, Koslowski, & Main, 1974).

Juxtaposed against this awareness of the expected maternal reaction to praise for one's child is the memory that my mother never said, "I'm proud of you." There was instead an abiding and implicit message that what I was doing was good and acceptable and expected. Praise for specific acts was unnecessary. I was always encouraged to "do your best." Correction was always muted, indirect, and often wordless, a glance or a shadow of disappointment falling quickly across my mother's or my grandmother's face.

I did know by my mother's quiet smile that she was proud of me. Yet, as a child, these quiet affirmations seemed inadequate, drowned out by the more seductive and lavish message of praise, praise, praise that sprang forth from the idealized visions of the parent–child relationship in the movies, on television, and in the books I read. These visions made my mother's affirmation of me seem insubstantial and without the conviction that rang so resoundingly in the proud statements made by the parents of my friends.

So, although I must labor to put aside my sense that danger lurks in acknowledging my children's individuality and spontaneity, I tell my children often that I feel proud of them, hoping that they can then be freed, as I was not, to "hear" too their mother's happiness, pleasure, and love in the spaces between the words.


## CONCLUSION

As I have worked to articulate fragments of encounters with myself as a mother and the mothering that I have received, I am left to ponder whether my efforts to bridge the cultural traditions joined within our family have entailed adopting a voice that turns away from the power of the unspoken, turns away from the assumption that you are known to the other as surely as you are known to yourself, and turns away from a moral vision in which the subordination of the self to the collectivity can bring a sense of well-being and maturity. I am certain these concerns will form the ongoing subtext of my motherhood, and that I will be searching for moments with my children that shield me from the losses inherent in our distance from my cultural tradition. I am therefore grateful to those who encourage me to trust that my children *will* find their way through the tangle of memories and convictions I hold dear and the ones I have adopted on their behalf, and still see me.

To conclude, and at the risk of sounding only like a proud mother, I share one final anecdote. It is an important touchstone as I nurture such trust in my children and myself. Eliza's teacher writes on her report card: "Eliza makes me smile. She is a friend to all, truly loving and concerned about others. She demonstrates a remarkable sensitivity to the feelings of others and is often instrumental in the resolution of conflict. She is enthusiastic, self-motivated, and proud of her accomplishments, yet is also able to be genuinely pleased by the achievements of her classmates." I was smiling and crying as I read this. I am certain my mother and grandmothers are smiling, too.

## REFERENCES

Anzaldua, G. (1987). *Borderlands/LaFrontera.* San Francisco: Spinsters/Aunt Lute.

Azuma, H. (1986). Why study child development in Japan? In H. Stevenson, H. Azuma, & K. Hakuta (Eds.), *Child development and education in Japan* (pp. 3–12). New York: Freeman.

Barnlund, D. C. (1975). *Public and private self in Japan and the United States.* Tokyo: Simul Press.

Benedict, R. (1946). *The chrysanthemum and sword.* Boston: Houghton Mifflin.

Benkov, L. (1994). *Reinventing the family: The emerging story of lesbian and gay parents.* New York: Crown.

Brazelton, T. B., Koslowski, B., & Main, M. (1974). The origins of reciprocity. In M. Lewis & L. Rosenblum (Eds.), *The effect of the infant on its caregiver* (pp. 46–76). New York: Wiley.

Caudill, W., & Weinstein, H. (1969). Maternal care and infant behavior in Japan and America. *Psychiatry, 32,* 12–43.

Cheung, K.-K. (1993). *Articulate silences: Hisaye Yamamoto, Maxine Hong Kingston, Joy Kogawa.* Ithaca, NY: Cornell University Press.

Clancy, P. (1986). The acquisition of communicative style in Japanese. In B. Schieffelin & B. Ochs (Eds.), *Language socialization across cultures* (pp. 213–250). New York: Cambridge University Press.

Conroy, M., Hess, R., Azuma, H., & Kashiwagi, K. (1980). Maternal strategies for regulating children's behavior: Japanese and American families. *Journal of Cross-Cultural Psychology, 11,* 153–172.

Doi, L. T. (1973). *The anatomy of dependence.* Tokyo: Kodansha.

Fogel, A., Stevenson, M. B., & Messinger, D. (1994). A comparison of the parent–child relationship in Japan and the United States. In J. L. Roopnarine & D. B. Carter (Eds.), *Parent–child socialization in diverse cultures* (pp. 35–51). Norwood, NJ: Ablex.

Hoefstede, G. (1991). *Cultures and organizations: Software of the mind.* London: McGraw-Hill.

Hoffman, E. (1989). *Lost in translation: A life in a new language.* New York: Penguin Books.

Hsu, F. L. K. (1981). *American and Chinese: Passage to differences.* Honolulu: University of Hawaii Press.

Kagitçibasi, C. (1990). Family and socialization in cross-cultural perspective. In F. Berman (Ed.), *Nebraska symposium on motivation* (pp. 135–200). Lincoln, NE: University of Nebraska Press.

Kagitçibashi, C. (1994). A critical appraisal of individualism and collectivism: Toward a new formulation. In U. Kim, H. C. Triandis, C. Kagitçibasi, S-C. Choi, & G. Yoon (Eds.), *Individualism and collectivism: Theory, method, and applications* (pp. 52–65). Thousand Oaks, CA: Sage.

Kogawa, J. (1981). *Obasan.* New York: Doubleday.

Kohlberg, L. (1969). *Stages in the development of moral thought and action.* New York: Holt.

Lebra, T. (1976). *Japanese patterns of behavior.* Honolulu: University of Hawaii Press.

Lebra, T. S. (1987). Silence in Japanese communication. *Multilingua, 6–4,* 343–357.

Markus, H. R., & Kitayama, S. (1991). Culture and the self: Implications for cognition, emotion and motivation. *Psychological Review, 98,* 224–253.

Markus, H. R., & Kitayama, S. (1994). The cultural construction of self and emotion: Implications for social behavior. In S. Kitayama & H. R. Markus (Eds.), *Emotion and culture: Empirical studies of mutual influence* (pp. 89–130). Washington, DC: American Psychological Association.

McLoyd, V. C. (1990). The impact of economic hardship on black families and children: Psychological distress, parenting and socioemotional development. *Child Development, 61,* 311–346.

Messinger, D. (1992). Autonomy and interdependence in Japanese and American mother–toddler dyads. *Early Development and Parenting, 1.*

Miller, J. G. (1994). Cultural diversity in the morality of caring: Individually-oriented versus duty-based interpersonal moral codes. *Cross-Cultural Research, 28,* 3–39.

Miyake, K., Campos, J., Kagan, J., & Bradshaw, D. L. (1986). Issues in socioemotional development. In H. Stevenson, H. Azuma, & K. Hakuta (Eds.), *Child development and education in Japan* (pp. 239–261). New York: Freeman.

Ruddick, S. (1989). *Maternal thinking: Toward a politics of peace.* Boston: Beacon Press.

Toda, S., Fogel, A., & Kawai, M. (1990). Maternal speech to three-month-old infants in the United States and Japan. *Journal of Child Language, 17,* 247–294.

Triandis, H. C. (1989). The self and social behavior in differing cultural contexts. *Psychological Review, 96,* 506–520.

Weingarten, K. (1997). *The mother's voice: Strengthening intimacy in families.* New York: Guilford Press. (Originally published 1994 by Harcourt Brace)

Weisz, J. R., Rothbaum, F. M., & Blackburn, T. C. (1984). Standing out and standing in: The psychology of control in America and Japan. *American Psychologist, 39,* 955–969.

Wierzbicka, A. (1991). Japanese key words and core cultural values. *Language in Society, 20,* 333–385.

Yeh, C. J. (1995). *A cultural perspective on independence in self and morality: A Japan and United States comparison.* Unpublished doctoral dissertation, Stanford University, Palo Alto, CA.

# 7

## He Needs His Father
### The Clinical Discourse and Politics of Single Mothering

*PHOEBE KAZDIN SCHNITZER*

### PROLOGUE

I am not a single mother, but for nearly 30 years, single-mother families have been at the center of my therapeutic, supervisory, and consulting activities. Early on, I became involved in a community-based clinical program of services to daycare and Head Start centers. The 10 years devoted to this program have been the most influential of my professional life, making it impossible for me to view child and family development in any way other than through the lens of social context. The single mothers I met, then and afterwards in outpatient work, taught me how families can overcome the restrictions and stigma perpetuated by public agencies and policy makers, as well as by some psychological theories and practice.

More recently, using the tools and language of narrative theories, I have been writing and speaking about single mothers, absent fathers, welfare, and the impact of poverty on mental health. It is my conviction that clinical practice, like other social phenomena, is best understood as a product of its time—influencing and influenced by the dominant social and political currents of the era. Clinical practice with single mothers and their children underlies all of this work; to these families I owe my greatest professional debt, and offer my greatest personal respect.

It is Thursday morning at the Thompson Day School. At 9:00 A.M. sharp, the teachers and clinicians begin to gather for this week's clinical progress conference. At this state-funded school for youngsters with behavioral problems and learning difficulties, each child's progress is subject to an annual review at which the academic, clinical, and administrative aspects of the treatment program are carefully considered. Today, Dr. T, a consulting psychiatrist, leads the discussion about a white, male adolescent, who entered the school a year and a half ago. Thirteen-year-old Patrick was referred to Thompson after he had been hospitalized for trying to throw himself in front of cars, saying and showing that he wanted to die. A sad child with subdued affect, he would occasionally bang his head—against a desk, once with a baseball bat—until he raised welts. When in public school, he didn't work, but played with plastic toys he'd bring with him.

Patrick is the younger of two boys being raised by a 35-year-old mother, Irene, who has been on her own since the boys were small. Patrick's father had been abusive to her, and she eventually asked him to leave. Out of touch for several years, this man reappeared to contact Patrick about 5 years ago, then vanished again. Prone to depression, Irene had given up her job in a nursing home and then, disabled by a painful orthopedic condition, had not been able to continue to care for the boys. After some time in foster care, both boys are now back with her. At the time of the conference, the family had recently been evicted from their apartment. Housed in a welfare motel, mother and two teenagers share a single room and cook off a hot plate. Miraculously, Patrick now shows up in school with his homework done and is able to do his classwork. Although looking less depressed, he is beginning to dabble in drugs and group delinquencies: A recent incident of vandalism landed him in court and earned him a probationary status.

After hearing this update, the consultant asks, "What about the father?" There isn't a lot known about him, just the history of abuse, and his erratic appearance and disappearance from Patrick's life. Irene has mentioned he may be in town; she thinks he's living with another woman and her children. "Does he see his son?" asks the consultant. There is a brief reiteration of the history, putting together that it was following his father's abrupt departure 5 years ago that Patrick became suicidal. Dr. T elaborates the risks for an adolescent boy being raised by a single mother without the father in the picture: greater antisocial involvement, poorer academic achievement, and low self-esteem, all related to his chronic "father hunger."

"What can we do to get this father in? How can we get him

involved?" the consultant asks. Mother's social worker reiterates the history of abuse, and that Irene, having struggled to get him out of the house, has no interest in reviving the relationship. Irene has been adamant that any renewed contact between Patrick and his father would have to be consistent, given her son's life-threatening response to his father's previous departure. "She's gatekeeping!" announces the consultant, who goes on to explain, "These mothers are the gatekeepers of contact between father and son; her own needs may be getting in the way of her hearing her child's need. Nothing is going to move in this case until the father gets more involved." In response to a dismaying array of issues—the housing crisis, mother's depression, Patrick's possible drug experimentation, increasing delinquencies, and the involvement of the court system—a summary is offered, a recommendation made: "Get the father in. He needs his father."

Of course Patrick needs his father, doesn't he? How could it be otherwise? But when clinicians decide what a child or a family needs, we are making interpretations that are influenced by our perceptions of *who* is needy, our formulations of *why* they are needy, and our (often foregone) conclusions about what constitutes a nonneedy situation. These perceptions, formulations, and conclusions about what is needed do not occur in a vacuum; they are intimately linked to the prevalent sociopolitical discourse of the times (Fraser, 1989). These links become apparent when we consider the possible meanings of the interpretation that "he needs his father," so often made when clinicians see families in which mothers are raising children on their own. Examining this particular clinical interpretation will then help us to approach the broader question of how clinical interpretations generally may reflect the socioeconomic and political contexts in which they occur.

This chapter begins with five vignettes from clinical practice and consultation, illustrating interpretations of need for the father that are commonly made by clinicians and parents alike. The examples all focus on single mothers raising sons, as it is particularly with regard to boys that this need is most urgently described. Although there is recognition in both popular and professional literature that fathers play crucial roles in young girls' development (e.g., Herzog, 1992; Hetherington, 1972, 1989; Secunda, 1992; Simpson, 1992), the social and clinical discourse elaborating the young girl's need for her father does not duplicate the sense of urgency for the developmental fate of the fatherless young boy. It is not within the scope of this discussion to explore fully the reasons for this contrast in discourse, whether it stems from perceived advantages that the little girl experiences in being raised by a same-sex parent, or from a perceived destiny of disadvantage, as an adult whose role is constrained by those very limitations from which her brother must be protected. But the contrast hints at the connection between the interpretation "he needs his father" and perceived deficiencies in the mothering role that are a central focus of this chapter. To explore this connection, I will examine how our national discourse depicts single mothers. From this specific question, I will turn to a general consideration of how sociopolitical discourse and clinical discourse may interrelate. Finally, I will revisit and elaborate the clinical material to consider paths by which mental health professionals might confront and resist the dominant clinical and social discourses in the domain of single mothering.

## INTERPRETING WHAT IS NEEDED

The following vignettes, derived from my clinical work and consultation, illustrate five components of a boy's need for his father: self-esteem, discipline, gender identity, supervision, and financial support. Discussion of these illustrations points up the ambiguity of what "need for the father" means in single-mother families, and suggests that it is in these domains that the mother's role is seen as most deficient. The examples show how perceptions of deficiency form the basis for personal behaviors and social interactions. In this way, the process of marginalization of single mothers—imposed by either self or society—occurs.

### Self-Esteem

On entering the Head Start classroom, I see 3- and 4-year-olds seated in a circle around their teacher for a singing game designed to help them learn each others' names. Each child is to say his or her name; then the whole group will sing the name several times. The teacher begins, saying her first name and her last name clearly for the children to repeat. As their turns come, some children follow her example, but others give only their first names, look down or away from the group, or mumble too softly to be heard. I don't understand why some children look so uncomfortable and say just their first names. In response to my confusion, the community social worker offers this explanation: Those children don't have fathers.

### Discipline

Fourteen-year-old Cormac has been caught shoplifting on several occasions; he has spent many hours doing community service, only to revert again to stealing cigarettes and toys from local shops. Cormac's dad is notified of his son's most recent court appearance and, despite a long previous absence from the family, joins Cormac and his mother at the hearing. The judge proposes a plan, whereby Cormac will accompany his father to work on Saturdays, earning spending money if he shows responsibility and follows directions.

### Gender Identity

Eight-year-old Damion had run, terrified, away from a neighborhood fight. Reaching home and finding his door locked, he had crawled in a window to safety. When his older sister found him hiding in a closet, she threw him outside and locked the door, saying he had to learn to fight. Describing this incident, his mother asks her social worker if Damion is going to grow up gay, because he only has women around him.

### Supervision

Although 10-year-old Freddie didn't get into real trouble, he kept his working mother busy with his demands. When she started to date a man from work, Freddie acted up, until his mother decided to call his dad, who lives out of state, has remarried, and has infrequent contact with the family. She explains that, on many days, Freddie is not where he should be after school, that he is staying out longer than she likes. Freddie's dad responds by inviting him up for a weekend.

### Financial Support

Ian's eighth birthday is coming up, and he has his eye on a much-needed pair of track shoes. His mother explains she can't afford them. She tells him if he wants them so badly, he can get on the phone and call his father, with whom neither he nor she has had any contact, not to mention child-support payments, in over a year. Despite his angry feelings toward his father, Ian calls and makes his request.

These examples, drawn from one biracial, one black, and three white family situations, illustrate some of the most widely accepted components of the male child's need for his father: He needs his father to establish self-worth and social standing; to help develop inner controls and gender identity; to rely on for supervision and finances. But it is virtually impossible to tease apart, in the examples above, whose needs are at stake. When Ian needs money, or Freddie needs supervision, are we noting the child's deprivation or the mother's financial and time constraints? When Cormac needs discipline do we deplore his lack of inner control or his mother's difficulty in controlling him by setting limits? Who is concerned that overexposure to women may lead to male homosexuality, the child, the mother, or "society"? When we assert that "he needs his father" in these ways, we are also implying that his mother cannot provide these things.

Of course, it is hard going for her to do it all, alone. The obvious answer, that both caretaker and child are needy, is ultimately the most meaningful in practical terms. But, this "obvious answer" may also obscure certain assumptions we hold about the role of provider and about controls, aggression, and male sexuality, of which male figures are often presumed to be in charge. We tend to assume that mothers are inadequate to these tasks (Silverstein & Rashbaum, 1994; Blankenhorn, 1995).

If the boy is to be properly raised, and the mother can't do it, then we had better get the father in to save the day, or at least to help out. But trying to solve the problem that way makes it harder to see that something else is being neglected: an adequate understanding of the mother's own needs and capabilities, as head of a single-parent family. Instead of asserting that "he needs his father," we might sharpen our focus and ask, "What do we think single mothers need to raise their children successfully?" Reflecting on the possible responses to this question makes clear that social and economic influences are at work. How the single mother is depicted—the images of who she is and what she needs, are intensely politicized issues.

## WHO IS THE SINGLE MOTHER?

Endless writings and media events have reiterated the debates on who the single mother is, and whether she needs the carrot or the stick to make a go of her life (Buckley, 1994; *Oprah,* 1994; Whitehead, 1993). With the 1996 passage of welfare reform, state and national policies have consolidated an answer: The single mother is a freeloader who must be made to work, a baby machine whose childbearing aspirations must be "capped"; an incompetent parent who must be prodded to keep her children in school. Between 1992 and 1995, when states were granted permission to test out welfare reforms, "workfare" require-ments were imposed in 28 states. Family "caps," denying benefits for any child born to a welfare recipient, were imposed by 18 states. Plans to deny aid to families whose children were truant (called "Learnfare") were approved in 25 states (Albelda, Folbre, & The Center for Popular Economics, 1996; A. Collins & Aber, 1996), despite the fact that research has found no difference in school attendance for children of welfare versus nonwelfare families (Rabinovitz, 1996).

The images of the single mother that pervade the media often focus on the overall rise in nonmarital births, the rise in nonmarital births to teenagers, and these proportions within the black population in particular. Startling statistics abound, but are rarely examined closely. For statistics, unlike the quality of mercy, do not drop from Heaven, but are calculated to highlight and inflame specific arguments. The intuitive sense that numbers are objective obscures the social reality that numbers are generated from within different ideological perspec-tives and are sometimes aimed at supporting specific social agendas (Crossen, 1994).

Statistical portraits of single mothers are provocative in several ways. A sensible first step for any interested researcher might be simply to describe who single mothers are in terms of demographic charac-teristics such as age, number of children, reason for being single, and income level. But data on these characteristics are not typically reported as proportions of the total single-mother population. For example, the U.S. Census Bureau's Reports on Household and Family Characteristics (1990) are organized to highlight racial and ethnic comparisons, making it easy to find that 19% of white families are headed by single mothers, in contrast to 29% of Hispanic families, and 56% of black families. Such presentations of data promote the widespread image of the typical single mother as an unmarried black woman, frequently portrayed as a teenager on welfare. Comparative data like these draw attention away from the fact that nearly two-thirds (65%) of all single mothers are white, that their median age is 33 years old, and that 81% of all single mothers have only one or two children (Center on Hunger, Poverty and Nutrition Policy, 1995). Furthermore, it is divorce and separation that account for most children living in single-mother families, not nonmarriage. Finally, only about one-quarter of single mothers are on welfare, while nearly half of all single-mother families live in poverty. In 1994, these families made up 39% of the homeless population (Albelda et al., 1996).

In contrast to presentations of data that highlight comparisons among subgroups of single mothers, other data tend to blur significant group distinctions: Most common is the blurring of boundaries between the total populations of single mothers, welfare *mothers,* and welfare *recipients.* Where distinctions are not clearly stated, these groups tend to be confounded, until it seems that all single mothers are on welfare, and all welfare recipients are single mothers. Sociologist Mark Rank (1994) has emphasized that single mothers are only one group of welfare recipients among several others: single (nonparent) adults; elderly persons; married couples; and single fathers. According to his Wisconsin sample, single mothers constituted just about 30% of all households entering the welfare system.

Going beyond the presentation of statistics, their interpretation is yet another source of ambiguity. Although demographers agree on the overall rise in single mothers, there is little consensus as to how to understand the increase (Bumpass, 1990). One alternative to a focus on birth rates is a focus on marriage and the reasons for its decline (Popenoe, 1996). Data from the U.S. Bureau of the Census (1993) show that there are nearly twice as many unmarried adults now as there were 20 years ago. Researchers such as William Julius Wilson (1996) and Frances Fox Piven (Piven & Cloward, 1993) have examined the decline in marriage from an economic perspective, and suggest that the single mother is one consequence of shifts in the economy. Availability of low-paying service sector jobs may increase women's economic independence. At the same time, the loss of better-paying jobs in manufacturing may shrink the market of marriageable men, particularly of black males (Wilson, 1996).

Economic instability is not the only possible factor underlying the decline in marriage rates. Soaring divorce rates, now at 60% of first marriages, are a familiar fact of life. One of the impacts of this widespread marital disruption may be that fewer people expect marriages to last; therefore, more people marry later or not at all. These competing explanations point up, at the very least, that there are many different reasons for being a single mother. Lesbian couples have shown an upsurge in motherhood, a lesbian baby-boom (Benkov, 1994). And many young, unmarried black women may be socialized to single motherhood by the successful experience of their mothers and older sisters (Williams, 1991).

But it is not only lesbian mothers and black women who are expressing the choice of going it "alone"; there are well-documented increases in single motherhood internationally. In attempting to understand this worldwide phenomenon, Australian researchers Ailsa Burns and Cath Scott review a variety of explanations and conclude that there is most support for "de-complementary" theories that recognize that the interests of women and men have become less interdependent. Alternatives to marriage become increasingly attractive as "men are likely to find family commitments too burdensome, and women are likely to find men and their requirements a burden" (1994, p. 185).

In contemporary American discourse, then, the diversity among single mothers and the possible reasons for their increase are entirely lost in the political fray. Because clinicians focus intently on individuals, they will obviously grasp the particulars of a single mother's past and present situation. But the negative national climate may increase the clinician's concerns about outcomes for single-mother families. Certainly the study of father absence has appeared more frequently in the last few years as the subject of books, articles, and conferences (e.g., Blankenhorn, 1995; Griswold, 1993; Phares, 1996; Popenoe, 1996; Snarey, 1993). How does this atmosphere of heightened concern—the combination of negative imagery of single mothers with intensified interest in absent fathers—influence the clinical treatment of single-mother families?

## CLINICAL INTERPRETATION IN POLITICAL CONTEXT

Any fantasy that the mental health professions operate independently of social context has surely been demolished by the transformations in treatment brought about by insurance requirements: the authorization of and response to client need are being substantially influenced by financial considerations. This is only one of many arenas in which we openly acknowledge that clinical interpretation occurs, not with the pristine objectivity naively associated with the "hard" sciences or medicine, but in all-too-humanly constructed social contexts that vary with innumerable historical, economic, and sociopolitical factors. We now acknowledge fairly comfortably that Freud's views of his female clients—their sexuality and symptomatology—were influenced by the Vienna of the 1900s. We acknowledge that interpretations and disclosures of sexual abuse are now more frequent because of the social climate of acceptance of these phenomena.

It is always easier to see in retrospect how economic and political factors have influenced sociocultural issues, including psychological formulations in the area of single mothering. A historical focus on topics related to single mothering yields compelling illustrations of salient economic and political influences. For example, changes in the labor market, accompanied by an expansion or contraction of welfare benefits, may influence how single mothers on welfare are depicted. Summarizing their historical survey of public relief, Piven and Cloward (1993) argue that the growth of low-paying jobs "requiring" cheap labor encourages cutbacks in welfare benefits: at these times, negative images of welfare recipients tend to increase. In a different vein, Solinger's study (1992) of adoption in the post-World War II era examined the pregnancy outcomes of black and white unwed mothers. White unwed mothers were described as misguided or neurotic and in need of help to relinquish their infants and get back on track. Black single mothers were described as intentionally having intercourse, desiring motherhood, and therefore wanting to keep their babies. These young women's psychological profiles appeared to correlate with different adoption demands for black versus white babies. Finally, psychological research on effects of father absence also appears to vary with the social and political climate (McLanahan & Booth, 1989). The questions asked and the conclusions drawn have shifted, from a post-World War II documentation of devastating effects of father absence, through a more "liberal" period during the 1960s and '70s, of optimistic identification of factors supporting single-mother success; back to a contemporary, conservative focus on the wide-ranging ills we can expect when a child is raised by a mother alone (Schnitzer, 1993).

Historical perspectives facilitate our understanding of influential social and political contexts; it is harder to see how current sociopolitical influences operate and possibly impact psychological interpretation. It is difficult, for example, to sort out the reciprocal influences on clinicians and by clinicians in the national fervor to bring fathers back to their family responsibilities. The relationship between views of mental health and dominant socioeconomic currents goes two ways.

On the one hand, mental health language may shape and support the national social discourse. "Expert" vocabularies and rhetoric, such as those used by lawyers or psychotherapists, tend to bridge social phenomena and government policy making. The identification of needs in professional language such as "paternal deprivation" or "father hunger" may pave the way for social and economic hardship to be construed as social or psychological deviancy. Government policy is then framed to provide social, not economic, responses (Fraser, 1989).

It is also apparent that socioeconomic issues may influence definitions of mental health. There is now strong agreement that poverty increases stress and depression (Desjarlais, Eisenberg, Good, & Klerman, 1995; Schnitzer, 1996); some channels by which poverty makes this impact on women include dangerous neighborhoods, housing problems, and undermined social relationships (Belle, 1990). Nearly half of single-mother families live in poverty or are homeless: Do clinicians sometimes "therapize" conditions ultimately stemming from inadequate income, housing, and supervision, by diagnosing "father hunger," as Dr. T did in the opening vignette?

It is not, however, simply a matter of what clinicians choose to see and treat. Social influences affect both therapists and clients. Many a single mother experiences herself as incapable of raising a child alone, particularly if that child is a son; indeed, family therapists have noted how single mothers may see therapy as a way to heal the "incompleteness" of their family, or to correct their ineffective or incompetent handling of sons (Morawetz & Walker, 1984; Sheinberg & Penn, 1991). The mother described above, who thought she was promoting homosexuality in her son, requested a male therapist to help him learn to fight. Therapists and clients might usefully explore together how child and family problems come to be identified as needing mental health intervention, as opposed to other forms of help.

The decision that a given situation calls for psychotherapy presumably is made in the course of a diagnostic evaluation; but that decision may ultimately depend on the conscious and unconscious mix of political agenda with clinical understanding—not to mention the economic needs of therapists, issues with which clinicians are typically uncomfortable. As critical theorist Edward E. Sampson writes, "Our traditional science has taught us that the psychological must be separated from the political" (1993, p. 1228). Closely examining our assumptions is one way to begin to broach whatever biases may be embedded in our clinical outlooks.

Two provocative challenges to assumptions about single mothering illustrate what some clinicians may currently be taking for granted. First of all, when is a father really absent? Physical residence in the home is only one way a father may be present in his child's life; "absent" black fathers are more likely than their white counterparts to live nearby, to be present occasionally, and to visit frequently or in times of emergency (Mott, 1990; E. Sparks, personal communication, June 3, 1994).

A second challenge has been raised to mainstream assumptions about the proper timing of pregnancy, assumptions held by many clinicians as well. Noting in a 1989 interview that everybody's grandmother was a teenager when they got pregnant, Nobel prize-winning author Toni Morrison exclaimed, "Who cares about the schedule? What is this business that you have to finish school at 18?" (Taylor-Guthrie, 1994, p. 260). The timing of major events in the lives of teenage girls may be transmitted by powerful subcultural norms, constituting a "teen Mommy track" (Hymowitz, 1994). This challenge to ideas about the "right order" for one's life script is supported by the findings that increasing numbers of women are reentering formal education after a hiatus (Scarbrough, 1994), and therefore not losing out educationally because they have had their children first.

These challenges to mainstream assumptions clearly have the status of marginal, not dominant discourse. The primary purpose they serve here is to highlight what clinicians may take for granted about single mothering, and to spur on the process of making explicit the ideologies that underlie clinical interpretations.

## REVISITING NEED: ALTERNATE VIEWS

The clinical vignettes presented initially illustrated five commonly proposed components of the male child's need for his father: self-esteem, discipline, gender identity, supervision, and financial support. Interpreting problems in these areas as evidence of a boy's "paternal hunger" is consistent with an ideology that sees single-mother households as failed family structures that should be corrected primarily by moving the fathers back into the picture. We have examined how statistical portrayals of single mothers simultaneously express and reinforce the dominant negative social biases about single-mother families. And, in discussing the interrelationship of national discourse and clinical discourse, we have noted how difficult it can be for mental health professionals to recognize the embeddedness of clinical interpretation in current sociopolitical contexts. Becoming aware of assumptions that influence the interpretation of need in single-mother families would, ideally, include realization of the actual diversity among single mothers and recognition that a focus on absent dads tends to narrow perceptions of present moms to a stereotype of inherent incapability. It is this damaging stereotype that clinicians can confront and resist in a variety of ways. Instead of prioritizing "getting the father in," clinicians can focus on strengthening the mother's competencies, clarifying the distinctions between her needs and the needs of her child, and taking both into account in responding to the family. There is no reason to assume that getting the father in is an aim that excludes any of this work; however, it may well be that the priorities the therapist conveys to the mother, with implications about her general competency and her specific ability to raise a son, make an important impact. Similarly, when her son sees that his mother is respected as a caretaker and is fully expected to be in charge of her family, he, too, may increase his security and confidence that his family will be all right.

In revisiting the five vignettes with which this chapter began, we will explore more extensively certain clinical issues that might be glossed over by a too-rapid formulation of "father hunger." In this way, we can see the possibilities for clinical conversations other than "he needs his father." By resisting and opposing the narrowed perceptions of single mothers and exploring expanded possibilities for action, the process of marginalization can be reversed, at least within the domain of the clinical hour. Resistance to stigmatizing perceptions precedes and provides the foundation for resistance to marginalizing actions by the mother herself.

## Self-Esteem: Shame Versus the Need to Know

The first vignette, about youngsters supposedly too ashamed to say their names implies automatic attribution to all father-absent children of the opprobrium traditionally associated with out-of-wedlock child-bearing. Shame about father absence is not automatic, but is taught to children by the behavior of those around them, such as a hesitancy to allow open communication on the subject. In the absence of permission to ask questions or clarify why the family is the way it is, children may become generally uncertain about what they think, feel, or do.

"Something's missing"—a father-absent youngster began every session by announcing, on entering the therapy room, that "something's missing, something's different." With chronic sadness, this 8-year-old faced his day with a sense of loss he could not readily identify. Not understanding one critical absence, all things became potentially absent-able. In his confusion, he carried with him fears that others would leave, fears of abandonment, and a chronic sense of something "not right."

In her 1992 novel *Jazz,* Toni Morrison likens the absent father to a missing limb and discusses the need to know: "I am not angry, I don't need the arm. But I do need to know what it would have been like to have had it. . . . It's a phantom I have to behold. . . . Will it even know who or what I am? It doesn't matter. . . . I will locate it so the severed part can remember the snatch, the slice of its disfigurement. Perhaps then the arm will no longer be a phantom, but will take its own shape, grow its own muscle and bone" (p. 159).

The need to know, inseparable from the pain of loss, may be the major factor in the mastery of that pain. I am proposing that a crucial component of the child's self-esteem is cognitive: the confidence that one is able to make sense of one's world. Children raised by single mothers will need to understand what happened to their father, the story of his one-time presence and of his present absence. Self-esteem is strengthened and shame is countered by cognitive clarity over what happened.

Clinicians can facilitate such conversations in therapy with mother and child together. But stories of why the father is absent, what he was like, what is currently known about him often present dilemmas for both clients and therapists, particularly when young children are involved. The therapeutic challenge comes from impulses to shield children from potentially damaging visions of adult relationships. When parents turn to family therapy for help in telling children about traumatic events, the work might involve reviewing multiple versions: What does the mother believe about the father's absence? What has she already said to her children, and to other family members and friends? What does she fear if certain details were disclosed? The child, also, will hold multiple versions of his parents' relationship: snatches of gossip picked up in the neighborhood, explanations from the father himself on a previous visit or in a letter or phone call, or fantasies elaborated from television images or personal longings. Attending to the range of parental and child renditions of what happened in their family demonstrates that these matters are open for discussion, not closed by shame (Schnitzer, 1993).

## Discipline: Helping Mothers Set Limits

There are numerous ways in which clinicians can help mothers with limit setting, ranging from formal behavioral modification programs to informal agreements about consequences. What stands in the way is not so much the means, but the lack of conviction about the mother's effectiveness. It is not a matter of women not being able to set limits; we question what would happen if mothers were to discipline sons too well. There is a long tradition in this country, dating from at least the period of World War II, which insists that mothers can destroy manliness, that too much "listening to mother" produces feminized men (Griswold, 1993).

This fear of maternal overcontrol may be heightened in single-mother families. As a result, single mothers may end up exerting weaker controls and making fewer demands on their children than mothers who live with another adult family member (Dornbusch et al., 1985). It is not at all clear, however, that it is single mothers in particular who have this difficulty setting limits. Both male and female single parents have been found to report less restrictive rules than did married parents; every type of two-adult family, with the exception of mother–male-partner families, reported stronger controls than single-parent families (Thomson, McLanahan, & Curtin, 1992). Thus, interpersonal support for adequate behavior control by mothers may make a substantial impact.

Cormac's father, as described above, was called upon by the judge to take Cormac to work for 6 months to earn money to pay off what he had stolen. This arrangement lasted two weekends. Ultimately, it was Cormac and his mother who sat down with their family therapist and the state's Department of Social Service Worker to seek out a summer job, and discuss the daily obligations on Cormac to be more responsible, and the consequences if he was irresponsible. Though initially tentative, Cormac's mother gained confidence and was eventually able to implement their plan with good results.

## Gender Identity

Closely related to the fears about maternal discipline are vague notions that too much womanly contact produces homosexuality. Even within two-parent families, a close relationship between mother and son may be seen as suspect for "unhealthy" development (Sheinberg & Penn, 1991). But theorists such as Pollack and Grossman (1985) and Herzog (1992) suggest that important affective qualities may be learned or enhanced by intimate involvements with women, and that these qualities constitute strengths, not weakness.

Even less admissible than fears of homosexuality are fears of mother–son incest in single-mother households. Unspoken sexual tensions may drive mothers and teenage sons into battle. Clinicians tend to view sexualized behaviors with alarm, calling any affectionate display into question as seduction. The urgency to separate mother and son, and to insist on the need for a male presence in their midst, may derive in part from nonexplicit notions of protecting the son from the mother's seductiveness and protecting the mother from the son's sexual approach. The distinctions between physical affection and sexualized physical contact, and their positive and/or negative impacts, remain undertheorized and underresearched areas.

One of the derivatives of this concern about seductiveness may be the idea, held by both parents and clinicians, that boys should discuss sexual matters with men, not women.

Damion's mother and older sister both feared he might grow up to be gay because of their influence on him. The mother's social worker didn't feel she knew very much about causes of homosexuality, so she decided to educate herself as best she could with consultation on the subject, which she then introduced into the therapy. In the course of this discussion, Damion's mother mentioned that his older sister had recently revealed she was a lesbian. The mother's dismay and guilt, and her fears about homosexuality in both men and women were then explored. It later emerged that Damion spied on his mother when she was changing her clothes. The therapist talked with mother and son about adults and children respecting each other's privacy, about their ideas about sex, and about questions they each had. Damion's mother began to realize she could address her son's sexual concerns, even though she wasn't male.

In contrast to self-esteem, inner controls, and gender identity, supervision and financial support are not psychological variables, but pertain more to structural aspects of the family environment. But supervision and financial support have significant psychological ramifications for the child and can usefully be discussed in therapy.

### Supervision

Adequate daycare and afterschool programs do not exist in this country, and the demand placed on single mothers to make arrangements for supervision is not always understood or viewed sympathetically.

When 7-year-old Jamie told his teacher that he had "lots of mothers," she was concerned, and thought he was showing signs of confused thought processes, reflecting his unstable chaotic family environment.

The idea of "other mother," described by Patricia Hill Collins

(1991), calls attention to the tradition of sharing mothering responsibilities in African American communities. "Other mothering" may mean that children spend significant amounts of time in households other than that of their biological mother, ranging from temporary childcare arrangements to long-term care or even informal adoptions. When viewed from the perspective of the mythologized white, middle-class, intact family, these arrangements may seem predominantly chaotic, and their adaptive aspects overlooked.

It turned out that Jamie often spent weekends with his grandmother, and that he also had a young aunt who took him out regularly, which Jamie viewed as a special treat. Jamie's mother was trying to take some courses, and particularly when she had papers due, she relied heavily on her family to take care of her children. In therapy, conversation reviewed Jamie's experiences with his extended family members and the reasons for his mother's busy schedule, as well as the advisability of the mother clarifying for Jamie's teacher the nature of his childcare arrangements. Providing physical security is not all there is to supervision; it is also a matter of providing the assurance of psychological presence.

As discussed at the outset, 10-year-old Freddie began acting up around the time his mother was beginning to date. The therapist speculated on the coincidence of Freddie's not being home and his mother's not being home. In family therapy, Freddie told his mother that he was worried that she would marry and have new babies, whom she would "love better" than him. His mother reassured him that she would always love him and explained that that was why she needed to know where he was in the afternoons. A telephone arrangement was established with Freddie calling his mother at work, to check in when he came home each day from school.

## Financial Support

Nearly half of all families headed by single mothers live in poverty, many of them as part of the homeless population. The effect on children of this economic insecurity has long been one of the central concerns about single mothering (McLanahan & Sandefur, 1994).

Children in single-parent homes are very likely to be aware of the precariousness of their family's financial state and are often caught in precisely the bind that is so intensely discussed on the national level: When money is tight, do you seek out (absent) Dad, or do you pressure (present) Mom to provide the goods? Many children learn that shared parental responsibility is unlikely. Instead they experience significant hardship, share the mother's struggles to make ends meet, and witness intense battles among adults over money.

The same child, Ian, who got on the phone to his father about track shoes, expressed multiple fears about his mother's capacity to earn and about what would happen to her job if he or she got sick. In conversations in family therapy, he voiced these fears to his mother, who talked to him in more detail about her job situation and about how his older sisters would help out in an emergency. Ian also expressed his anger about his father's lack of financial support, stating he wanted no further contact with his father. He let his mother know he didn't like getting on the phone with requests and would not do it again.

Therapists are more likely to be attuned to the psychological or metaphorical implications of finances, rather than the real-life role of money in families (Mellan, 1992). Advocating for financial resources, whether involving child-support collection, welfare, or subsidized housing, sometimes raises questions about a clinician's proper role and whether therapy should rightly include forms of activism (Gallagher, 1992). The relative status of in-the-office and out-of-the-office work and the professionals who do it is an old question; hierarchies exist in which higher-status traditional therapies focus more on individual attribution of problems, while less-recognized, innovative models are more likely to address social structure issues. Advocacy and consult-ation do the latter, and so do group therapies. Single-mothers' groups may discuss financial matters, such as budgeting or child-support collection, and also more fundamental issues of long-term earning potential. Group members who support each other in achieving high school equivalency or returning to higher education are working on critical elements in increasing a single mother's ability to support her family.

These expanded discussions of situations commonly evoking the view that the boy "needs his father" point to therapeutic strategies centering on the family members who are present: mother and child. By pursuing conversations in which the competency of the mother is enhanced, the viability of the single-mother-and-child household is strengthened. Clinicians can therefore avoid simply replaying in clini-cal language the widespread social message that single-mother families are failed social structures. The clinical interchange does not become just one more arena in which the dominant social discourse is reiter-ated, but instead becomes an opportunity for both client and clinician to develop an alternate vision of single mothering—and, perhaps, parenting in general.

## CONCLUSION

There are schools of thought that emphasize that the father per se is not what is "really" needed, that what we intend when we identify "father hunger" is to underscore the ideal functions the father role represents. This genre of argument goes in various directions: It is not the biological father that the child needs, but an adult male father figure. It is not the father-in-the-home he needs, but male contact, by way of visits or neighborhood presence. Sometimes the argument goes that it is not a father who is needed, but an extra pair of hands, the offer of help and support being just as useful if it comes from a grandmother or aunt. Sometimes the argument goes that what the child needs is exposure to an adult dyad, to experience a triadic relationship.

I am troubled by these arguments, not because I think that mother and children are always fine on their own but because of the mode of analysis involved: basically see what's missing and try to replace it one way or another, like filling in for a missing puzzle piece with a cardboard substitute. These arguments miss something vital.

The focus on idealized father-functions ignores real-life men and real-life families. When we do "get the fathers in," clinicians learn pretty fast that their mere presence isn't going to fix everything. In the situations described above, Ian's and Freddie's fathers held steady jobs. But Cormac's father was an alcoholic who worked only sporadically and was in trouble with the law. Damion's father was a seriously ill diabetic, often hospitalized. Absent fathers, like single mothers, come in many varieties; if we do succeed in "getting the father in," we had better be prepared to hear his problems when he comes. Economic hardship, sometimes compounded by racial or ethnic discrimination, renders many fathers incapable of saving the day. For some, traumatic histories may be involved: Patrick's abusive father had been abused himself as a child. Clinicians may pin their hopes on the participation of an absent father, only to learn that his absence from the family may not be a problem but, rather, a solution.

Perhaps we should consider the possibility that the worldwide increases in single mothering express a growing intolerance for problematic implementations of marriage and family. Instead of accommodation, perhaps what is required is transformation. The idealized father-functions don't just need to be put back into the family, the family may need transformation to be a healthy, respectful, economically viable environment for all its members.

Single motherhood acts as a lightning rod, attracting political, social, economic, racial, and gender issues, ultimately revolving around the oldest of questions: *Who pays*—for childcare, child support, or job training; and *who's in charge*—of women's role definitions and reproductive rights. All families need to survive above the poverty line and find ways to balance breadwinning and caregiving. The growth of single-mother families is signaling that we need to transform family life, with rights and responsibilities balanced between partners and a more respected place for family supports in our national priorities.

## REFERENCES

Albelda, R., Folbre, N., & The Center for Popular Economics (1996). *The war on the poor: A defense manual.* New York: New Press.

Belle, D. (1990). Poverty and women's mental health. *American Psychologist, 45,* 385–389.

Benkov, L. (1994). *Reinventing the family: The emerging story of lesbian and gay parents.* New York: Crown.

Blankenhorn, D. (1995). *Fatherless America: Confronting our most urgent social problem.* New York: Basic Books.

Buckley, W. F. (1994, March 15). *A Firing Line debate resolved: Welfare has done more harm than good.* Columbia, SC: Producers Incorporated for Television.

Bumpass, L. L. (1990). What's happening to the family? Interactions between demographic and institutional change. *Demography, 27,* 483–498.

Burns, A., & Scott, C. (1994). *Mother-headed families and why they have increased.* Hillsdale, NJ: Erlbaum.

Center on Hunger, Poverty and Nutrition Policy. (1995). *Statement on key welfare reform issues: The empirical evidence.* Medford, MA: Tufts University.

Collins, A., & Aber, J. L. (1996). *State welfare waiver evaluation: Will they increase our understanding of the impact of welfare reform on children?* New York: National Center of Children in Poverty, Columbia University School of Public Health.

Collins, P. H. (1991). *Black feminist thought.* New York: Routledge.

Crossen, C. (1994). *Tainted truth: The manipulation of fact in America.* New York: Simon & Schuster.

Desjarlais, R., Eisenberg, L., Good, B., & Klerman, A. (1995). *World mental health: Problems and priorities in low-income countries.* New York: Oxford University Press.

Dornbusch, S. M., Carlsmith, J. M., Bushwall, S. J., Rittor, P. L., Leiderman,

H., Hastorf, A. H., & Gross, R. T. (1985). Single parents, extended households, and the control of adolescents. *Child Development, 56,* 326–341.

Fraser, N. (1989). Struggle over needs: Outline of a socialist–feminist critical theory of late-capitalist policy culture. In N. Fraser (Ed.), *Unruly practice: Power, discourse and gender in contemporary social theory* (pp. 161–187). Minneapolis: University of Minnesota Press.

Gallagher, N. (1992). Feeling the squeeze. *Family Therapy Networker, 16,* 16–29.

Griswold, R. I. (1993). *Fatherhood in America: A history.* New York: Basic Books.

Hetherington, M. (1972). Effects of father's absence on personality development in adolescent daughters. *Developmental Psychology, 7,* 313–326.

Hetherington, M. (1989). Coping with family transitions: Winners, losers, and survivors. *Child Development, 60,* 1–14.

Herzog, J. (1992). L'enseignement de la langue maternelle: Aspects du dialogue développemental fille-père. *Journal de la Psychanalyse de l'Enfant, 11,* 47–58.

Hymowitz, K. S. (1994, Autumn). The teen mommy track. *City Journal,* 19–29.

McLanahan, S., & Booth, K. (1989). Mother-only families: Problems, prospects, and politics. *Journal of Marriage and the Family, 51,* 557–580.

McLanahan, S., & Sandefur, G. (1994). *Growing up with a single parent: What hurts, what helps.* Cambridge, MA: Harvard University Press.

Mellan, O. (1992). The last taboo. *Family Therapy Networker, 16,* 40–47.

Morawetz, A., & Walker, G. (1984). *Brief therapy with single-parent families.* New York: Brunner/Mazel.

Morrison, T. (1992). *Jazz.* New York: Knopf.

Mott, F. L. (1990). When is a father really gone? Paternal–child contact in father-absent homes. *Demography, 27,* 499–517.

*Oprah.* (1994, January 19). I kicked welfare, you can too [transcript]. Livingston, NJ: Burrell's Information Services.

Phares, V. (1996). *Fathers and developmental psychopathology.* New York: Wiley.

Piven, F. F., & Cloward, R. A. (1993). *Regulating the poor: The functions of public welfare.* New York: Vintage.

Pollack, W. S., & Grossman, F. K. (1985). Parent–child interaction. In L. L'Abate (Ed.), *The handbook of family psychology and therapy* (Vol. 1, pp. 586–622). Homewood, IL: Dorsey Press.

Popenoe, D. (1996). *Life without father.* New York: Free Press.

Rabinovitz, J. (1996, May 7). Welfare cuts for truancy are stalled. *The New York Times,* p. B1.

Rank, M. (1994). *Living on the edge: Realities of welfare in America.* New York: Columbia University Press.

Sampson, E. E. (1993). Identity politics: Challenges to psychological understanding. *American Psychologist, 48,* 1219–1230.

Scarbrough, J. (1994). *Welfare women who pursue higher education: Transitions and transformations.* Unpublished manuscript.

Schnitzer, P. K. (1993). Tales of the absent father: Applying the "story" metaphor in family therapy. *Family Process, 32,* 441–458.

Schnitzer, P. K. (1996). "They don't come in!" Stories told, lessons taught about poor families in therapy. *American Journal of Orthopsychiatry, 66,* 572–582.

Secunda, V. (1992). *Women and their fathers.* New York: Delacorte Press.

Sheinberg, M., & Penn, P. (1991). Gender dilemmas, gender questions, and the gender mantra. *Journal of Marital and Family Therapy, 17,* 33–44.

Silverstein, O., & Rashbaum, B. (1994). *The courage to raise good men.* New York: Penguin.

Simpson, M. (1992). *The lost father.* New York: Knopf.

Snarey, J. (1993). *How fathers care for the next generation: A four-decade study.* Cambridge, MA: Harvard University Press.

Solinger, R. (1992). *Wake up little Susie: Single pregnancy and race before Roe v. Wade.* New York: Routledge.

Taylor-Guthrie, D. (Ed.). (1994). *Conversations with Toni Morrison.* Jackson, MS: University Press of Mississippi.

Thomson, E., McLanahan, S. S., & Curtin, R. B. (1992). Family structure, gender and parental socialization. *Journal of Marriage and the Family, 54,* 79–88.

U.S. Bureau of the Census. (1990). Household and family characteristics: March 1990 and 1989. In *Current population reports* (Series P-20, No. 447). Washington, DC: U.S. Government Printing Office.

U.S. Bureau of the Census. (1993). Marital status and living arrangements. In *Current population reports* (Series P-20, No. 468). Washington, DC: U.S. Government Printing Office.

Whitehead, B. D. (1993, April). Dan Quayle was right. *Atlantic Monthly,* pp. 47–84.

Williams, C. W. (1991). *Black teenage mothers: Pregnancy and child rearing from their perspective.* Lexington, MA: Lexington Books.

Wilson, W. J. (1996). *When work disappears: The world of the new urban poor.* New York: Knopf.

# 8

## Let Me Suffer So My Kids Won't

### African American Mothers Living with HIV/AIDS

KAREN FRASER WYCHE

*I* REMEMBER the first time I saw M. She was trying out an intervention study aimed at helping women living with AIDS and their teenage children communicate in more effective ways. I was the clinician who supervised the facilitators of the mothers and teen groups, though I had not attended one of their meetings before. I had come hoping to recruit some of the mothers for a small study I was starting in the future. Both M and I were visiting for the first time, but M was reluctant to be there. Her friend brought her saying that M was in denial about having AIDS. She was welcomed warmly by the other women, but she was shy. She was in her 40s, pudgy, short, and a beautiful color of chestnut brown, a woman who had been attractive before the drugs took over. Now in recovery and sick, she was not sure her youngest daughter would join the teen group that was part of the study. M had not been the best of mothers, and this daughter was angry.

Eventually, both mother and daughter joined the study groups. I continued to see M on videotapes of the group sessions that I viewed for supervision. From the safety of my living room, I watched M's physical decline as her illness progressed. She became thin, her skin became black and wrinkled, and her eyes sunken. Sometimes she was not in the group because she was hospitalized. When the interviewing for my study began, she said she was interested. But dementia had set in and she missed several appointments because of forgetfulness. I would call again and reschedule. I remembered what she said, "I haven't had anyone to talk to since the group ended." So, I kept rescheduling, knowing that she couldn't answer the questions I was going to ask. She finally came on a rainy, cold Saturday. Her daughter brought her. They were soaked. I made tea and gave her some rolls I had brought to share. She was very grateful. We sat together. She talked and I listened, for she could not understand the questions. She didn't remember we had both shared the first day of the group together. Soon after that meeting she died. She never realized that I had watched her for a year. I think of her and her fight with this terrible disease. I think of her daughter and her grandchildren. I see her face and hear her voice.

I have chosen M as the first woman to discuss in this chapter because her voice was silenced in so many ways by her illness, which resulted in dementia and then death. She represents the women who are diagnosed late in the course of their disease, when their illness progresses in ugly and predictable ways toward eventual death. The other women who speak in this chapter are living with AIDS. From their voices we learn of suffering and resistance to that suffering. They are mothers for whom the role of family is inextricably linked to their construction of their own reality within a cultural context. They are ill, poor, and African American. They struggle to maintain connections to their families and communities in the face of stigma and marginalization. But, before their stories can be told, it is important to know something about how the disease HIV/AIDS affects women.

## HIV/AIDS: WOMEN AND MOTHERS

Women are a vulnerable group in the HIV epidemic. The population of women who are diagnosed with HIV continues to grow, especially among African American women. The number of women who are at risk is also a concern of all health professionals. Several points are important for understanding the vulnerability of women to the AIDS epidemic.

1. Women are more likely to contract HIV through intravenous drug use contact than are men (Harverkos & Quinn, 1995).
2. Heterosexual transmission of HIV continues to grow, with women representing 38% of all reported AIDS cases (Centers for Disease Control and Prevention [CDC], 1996).
3. Women have a shorter survival time than men after diagnosis (CDC, 1997).
4. Minority women are overrepresented with AIDS, such that in 1991 27% of the AIDS diagnosed cases in women were white, 20% Latina, and 52% black (Ickovics & Rodin, 1992). By 1995, 77% of women diagnosed with AIDS were African American and Latina (CDC, 1996).
5. Large cities in the United States report a rise in the numbers of women who are becoming infected. For example, in New York City the percentage of AIDS cases in women increased from 12% in 1987 to 26% in 1993 (Maslanka, Lee, & Freudenberg, 1995).

For all racial minority women in the United States, who are disproportionately poor and have more children (Wyche, 1993), the disease presents major social and family problems. An infected mother of underage children is a serious problem because at present there is no cure for the disease. Decisions regarding custody of children loom in the background. This is a disease of concern to all women, not just minority women, because heterosexual transmission continues at a rapid rate, particularly among young women, and since 1985 the proportional yearly increase in death rate attributed to HIV infection in women has surpassed the death rate in men (CDC, 1997).

## MULTIPLE STIGMAS

Women who are diagnosed with HIV/AIDS, like those with other chronic diseases, live simultaneously in the medical and nonmedical communities. The medical community focuses on the body, the process of the disease, and ongoing changes in treatment approaches. For poor women, their medical community is the public clinic rather than the private practice office. They often experience gender discrimination, receiving fewer support services than many HIV/AIDS infected men, who may be included in well-developed networks of social services due to advocacy in the gay community (Hirshhorn, 1995).

Another community is the one in which minority women and their families live. For the African American women whose voices will be heard in this chapter, it is a community with chronic environmental stress. High crime rates, poor housing, densely populated neighborhoods, and low incomes combine to fill life with daily stress and challenge. Some of these women have left the drug community, which remains an ever-present force that could pull them back into its web. They have traded the community of illegal drugs that can kill them for the AIDS community of legal drugs to keep them alive longer.

Their simultaneous identities as members of deteriorating communities, racial minorities, and women, along with illness in general, combine to stigmatize and marginalize them. The negative stereotypes that are attached to these identities take on a new dimension when one has HIV/AIDS. The disease is stigmatizing. The view of people living with HIV/AIDS has been shaped by research and public health officials (Schiller, 1993): A degenerate gay culture of bath houses and prodigious numbers of sexual contacts and/or of addicts living in the streets sharing needles. This public idea of the "unworthy" people who contract HIV/AIDS also include mothers who are viewed as marginal—intravenous drug users or promiscuous—fit the public's view of the women who become infected. They are the ones society views as the "loose" women who are sexually deviant (Dora, Henderson, & South, 1994). It is not a view of mothers or grandmothers fulfilling the expected societal role for women as nurturers, or of women who chose the wrong man with whom to have unprotected sex. Women who are infected by partners whom they assume to be monogamous, regardless of their race or socioeconomic class, are not conceived of as belonging to this group. There are also women infected by heterosexual transmission from partners who have used intravenous drugs, rather than the women themselves being drug users (CDC, 1997). Few people can imagine that women over 50, mothers and grandmothers, are HIV positive, although we know that women of that age are often diagnosed in the later stages of the disease because physicians are not expecting to find them infected (CDC, 1997).

## STORIES OF MARGINALIZATION

The pathology model has been the traditional way minority women are described and/or studied by social scientists (Wyche, 1993), which of course also applies to African American women with HIV/AIDS. The term "minority" for the discussion here refers to those whom Ogbu (1988) describes as lacking in power (Native American, Latino, and African American) in the United States. The ways in which they are described go beyond mother blaming (see Introduction), which historically predominated in theoretical conceptions of white women. Instead, social science researchers tell stories with assumptions that maladaptive features exist in the behaviors and/or cognitions of people of color. Regarding African American women, topics of study are single parenthood, matriarchal family structures, teenage pregnancy, welfare dependency, or other such life conditions that result in problematic outcomes. Comparisons are made to European American, middle-class norms with resulting differences viewed as pathological and dysfunctional. There is no analysis of the structural racism, discrimination, and inequality that exist in the United States. No attempt is made to look at adaptive features of minority families, such as the role of kin and extended kin. The voice of minority mothers has not been heard in this professional/research discourse except in support of the pathology framework. The experience of these women is represented in ways that marginalize them rather than expressing or reflecting them. As a researcher/clinician who wants to understand the way women of color cope with HIV disease, this means I must resist the primary way they have been studied in this epidemic.

I wish to focus on what women tell me about their lives and how it relates to stress, coping, and daily survival. It is in keeping with the theme of this book to look at resistance to marginalization rather than psychological differences that divide women. We know that women describe both internal and external ways of coping with the dilemma of HIV/AIDS. Some studies that look at HIV-positive women have been prevalence studies of psychological distress with inappropriate comparisons made to men (Armistead & Forehead, 1995); many researchers who design intervention studies have been slow to realize that women are a special category. They are very different from gay men, who have been the focus of earlier work in this epidemic (Auerbach, Wypijewska, & Brodie, 1994). This focus is also characterized by researchers' generated variables. Lacking is the voice of the women in sharing their perceptions of the social influences and stress factors that may put them at risk. Personal narratives are not elicited to shape or change the intervention. When mothers are studied, it is typically with their children in cognitive behavioral interventions aimed at reducing parent–child conflict (Sherr, Hawkins, & Bennett, 1996).

We can ask the question of how mothers find ways to manage their lives when they are diagnosed with HIV disease. What are the life situations that they describe as stressful? How do they manage to cope with these situations? How does their role as a mother interact with these situations? How do they manage stigma? To answer these questions, I asked women to appraise their current life situation. This type of qualitative methodology was chosen because it allows women to tell me about the stress in their lives, how they cope with that stress, how social supports are utilized to mediate stress, and how culture mediates these outcomes.

## RESEARCH AS STORYTELLING

The reader should be very clear that all researchers choose the kind of story they wish their participants to tell. That is, they decide what the content of the story is going to be. This is called the hypothesis to be tested. They decide the characters of the story. The characters are called participants or subjects. The beginning of the story is the methodology, and the ending is the results. This ending occurs when the hypotheses are confirmed or not confirmed. Because most stories by researchers only get read when they are published in books or journals, the researchers look for ways to ensure that their story has the most likelihood of being read. As a result, the choice of the plot to develop the story or the theoretical framework becomes important.

So how can we study or tell a story about how women who share similar group characteristics (e.g., illness, ethnicity) live their lives? How can we study the cultural, social, and other ecological factors that impinge upon their lives and shape their behaviors? An interactive framework (Smith & Stewart, 1983) is the one that I use to tell the story I want in my research. There is no assumption that gender and race are homogeneous experiences. The focus is on distinct cultural values within groups. That is, what are the independent effects of experience that are uniquely defined by the individual? The other focus is on commonalities of experience across groups. To apply this framework to the study of the stress experienced by African American women who are diagnosed with HIV/AIDS, I ask a woman to tell me her story. This means asking her to define her experience and how that experience is related to stress and daily living, rather than assuming what her stress is and designing a methodology using researcher-generated variables of stress. By asking the woman first, I might discover aspects that I had not thought of investigating. So, if I want to study stress and parenting,

I might have some good guesses as to what the components of this might be from my clinical experiences and from the research literature. But, by asking the woman first, I might get information I had not expected, such as whether being a mother or a partner is more stressful. Or, whether being a member of a racial minority group and having a chronic fatal illness influences parenting. This approach listens to the voice of the woman and reports it. This approach to research includes the ecological or social context factors that contribute to risk, realizing that not everyone experiences risk in the same way.

But there are risks in this approach. Will the mothers I recruit for the study open up to me? As an African American woman will I, a college professor, be trusted even though I feel we are sisters? Will I remain faithful to their stories and report them accurately? I also feel another burden. The community in which these women live and receive medical care is also a community I lived in as a child. My feelings about this community are strong and positive. The hospital they come to for help also treated members of my family many years ago. Because so little maintenance has been done in the hospital all these many years, I can still find my way around. The walk from the subway to the clinic floods me with memories. I worry: Can I do the work, will I be true to the meaning of their words?

## THE STUDY

I designed a study that asked all the women to describe those aspects of their lives related to stress, coping, social support, and their health status. These are standard variables used in women's health research, especially related to cancer (Kurth, 1993; Sherr et al., 1996). The results discussed in this chapter are part of a larger qualitative and quantitative study in which I hope to understand how mothers experience stress in contexts that are beyond their control and how they invoke strategies to help deal with the resulting stress in their daily living.

The women you will read about were recruited from an infectious disease clinic in a large metropolitan hospital in New York City that serves primarily a low-income, Medicaid-patient population. All of the 14 women were African American and participated in a clinical trial that began in 1989. There were 17 women eligible for the study. However, one was incarcerated, one died, and the other could not be located. Eight of the women had tested positive for HIV, and six of the women had not. The HIV-negative women were seen for regular testing, however, because they were in a high-risk category for developing the disease—either they were intravenous drug users or had partners who were HIV-positive.

Women who have been monogamous with a partner and are not drug users usually are not distinguished by researchers from women who trade sex for drugs or who have been intravenous drug users. Many of those in the former category are unaware of the behaviors of their partners; the partners may have had other sexual partners (both male and female) who infected them and/or they may have engaged in drug use. For me these are the women whose faces and voices I remember most vividly from the interviews. They are truly victims because some did not suspect that their partners were engaged in high-risk behavior that would put them at risk.

This was not a group of young women. The mean age was 45 with a range of 36–62 years. Of the women, six had partners who had died of AIDS, five were currently in a relationship, and ten had children, ranging in age from 5 to 37. Because they were mothers at young ages, six of the women also had grandchildren. Most of the women were unemployed (80%) and had at least a high school diploma (72%).

I interviewed all of the women. The interview was a semistructured one that I had used previously with a different sample of women who had stressful lives (mothers of children who had mild to moderate retardation) (Wyche & Lobato, 1996). Thus, I knew that the questions elicited responses about the behaviors of interest regarding stress and coping (both adaptive and nonadaptive) and the cultural ways in which this happens. This previous work had indicated that the interview was sensitive to each woman's story. As a woman researcher, I was particularly concerned with trying to be respectful of these women who were doing me a favor by sitting for 2 to 2½ hours and telling their story to a stranger. I was particularly aware of the fact that these women had been recruited from a clinical trial where they were used to being questioned and examined every time they came into the clinic. For that reason, much of my time was spent explaining the study, answering questions, and trying to make each woman as comfortable as possible. Every woman received $25 for her participation. My experience was that the women were able to involve themselves in the interview and to feel safe. For example, several times I was asked for referral information regarding psychological counseling or other resources.

The specific questions were as follows: What kinds of things cause you stress? If you have a problem, who can you go to? Who can you get advice from? Who is concerned about you? Who can you talk to about feelings? What kind of help is available to you in your family? What strategies do you use to manage stress? Do you consider yourself a spiritual or religious person? In what ways does your religious or spiritual practice work for you in your life? Do you pray? How does prayer work for you in your life? How does your spiritual or religious life and your culture influence you as a woman? These questions were asked in a conversational way so that the questions and answers flowed together.

### Experiences of Mothering

These 14 women provide vivid accounts of the experience of mothering as a function of being either HIV-positive or HIV-negative. Some of the women were grandmothers, sisters, or took on a mothering role for other young women. The following discussion focuses on the themes that emerged.

#### Stigma

Many people who have the virus or the disease report that they fear discrimination ("felt stigma") and rejection by loved ones as well as acquaintances and strangers. They struggle to resist the stereotypes of "bad" and "unworthy," which create both socially or self-inflicted feelings of inferiority.

> "They don't want you around them because, see, like, if they don't understand about the virus, they think you can get it just being around you. This fellow told me that his mother found out that he had it and she put him out."

Another woman said:

> "The way they feel is, um, a curse, it's a punishment; a lot of people are heartless toward it and society looks at it that way, you know, people with the virus are either whores, they sleep around, or they use drugs."

These views of infected people thus interact with family dynamics. Naturally, people who are HIV-positive do not want to be rejected by their families or others, but these quotes show how clearly the women understand the stigma attached to HIV/AIDS, a stigma both frightening and unwanted.

## Connectedness/Disconnectedness with Children and Mothers

Finding out their HIV status turned out to be a pivotal situation that crystallized the relationships with their own children and mothers. The social status of being a mother takes on additional dimensions when the mother becomes diagnosed with a stigmatizing disease like HIV. When the women found out their test results, responses of joy and sadness revealed relationship issues with children or their own mothers.

A 44-year-old mother who tested negative said:

> "My kids were very glad. My grandchildren too. 'Cause everybody thought I had the disease. . . . My son and me are so much alike. Me and him probably worried together. Him in the Bronx, and me down here."

Women who were negative had been tested on a regular basis for several years. Coming to the clinic for these occasions brought out family issues. A 48-year-old HIV-negative woman stated:

> "My daughter, I always tell her I'm coming. I have two daughters, 24 and 21, and I tell them because I say, 'Well, I'm going to get my results,' and they like to know and stuff. My mother, she don't want to know. She don't want to hear about it, nothing. If you got a disease, she don't want to hear."

Relationships with their own mothers were often problematic regardless of diagnosis. Some women who were HIV-positive had had difficult times with both their mothers and their children. They are trying to resist psychological and relational disconnection that can impede development and threaten their psychological health.

A 38-year-old woman:

> "I'm gonna tell her. I don't know, it's just my mother's ways are funny . . . and it gets to me, so to avoid seeing her and being hurt. I can deal with it myself."

This quote shows a resistance to taking herself totally out of the relationship with her mother by silencing herself. This woman's conflict is vividly clear. She wants to tell her mother but anticipates that her mother will reject her ("her ways are funny"). So, to avoid being hurt by this, she will keep the secret and deal with it herself.

A 42-year-old woman on waiting 6 months to tell her daughter about her diagnosis:

> "I was ashamed because my mother always told me I would never amount to anything."

A 46-year-old grandmother said:

> "I dare not tell my kids [her sister knows], 'cause I don't know how they would act. I think my oldest son knows because him and my husband [who died of AIDS] were close, and I think he knows I have it, but I'm not sure. I got a funny feeling he knows but is just waitin' for me to come out and say it . . . I would never tell her [daughter] because she would treat me much different than now. I was hinting to her last Sunday and I said no, just leave it like it is. So, I said when the time comes, I'll tell her."

These women's emotional responses to informing children and family about their HIV status reveal connections and disconnections in families—the complexities of family relationships. They struggle with the "right" time to tell their story.

But some stories are happier, like this one from a 62-year-old grandmother:

> "My daughter took it. She said, 'Well, Mommy, don't worry. Things like that happen you know.' . . . And she said when her father died, . . . 'I have no one but you now.' "

These themes evidence a mixed response of support and stigma from mothers and children. Some are afraid of the possibility of disconnections from loved ones. Others are confident and connected. But, they all emphasize the relational past, present, and future. The women who did not get support were very sad over its absence as well as the real or potential break in embeddedness in family relations.

## Spirituality and the Protection of Children

The deep spiritual faith shared by these women came out in their feelings of protection for their children and grandchildren. They were not worried about themselves or focused on their illness. Not one woman spoke about wanting to have a cure for herself. They focused on others, especially their children and families, instead of themselves. They were not angry about their disease, but instead saw it as another chapter in their difficult lives. Their deep spirituality appeared to be a reason for these attitudes. Their spirituality could be seen as their strategy for resistance in the face of despair. Prayers for protection of children were common.

> "I just pray, you know, to make sure she's OK, 'cause she's 11 and tall as I am and she is developed, so I pray. She's in the building and, you know, the elevator and things like that. . . . I just say, please, Jesus, make sure she is OK, and this Sunday I'll do this and that . . . I'll read two pages of the Bible."

Or from another mother:

> "I ask God to let me go through the problems and things so they won't have to, sickness and things like that, 'cause I know what I went through with drugs and stuff. I don't want my kids to go through that. So let me suffer so they won't have to. And I believe that's what happened, because I've been suffering. But, it's easing up now, you know. I get well and go back in the hospital, like a year or 2 later for medicine and then back in . . . and you know I just ask to let me suffer so they won't have to. And I did, and they don't, and I'm happy about that. I think He's doing what I'm asking."

Women with adult children naturally focused on the youngest, the grandchildren.

> "I only ask God for my health and my strength to make sure that I live long enough to see my grands grow up and take care of my family, to take care of my friends and my enemies."

> "I thank God that I did grow up to see that I was able to have a daughter and grandkids and seeing them growing. . . . I feel good to be a woman."

Spirituality was also relied on to review where they were in their lives and how far they had come:

"I feel bad because I've used drugs and everything like that. I feel like God have forgiven me. It helps me because I can pray to him to protect my children . . . make my children safe from harm, and it just helps me."

The spirituality was focused on maintenance of their relations to others as well as to those who would survive them. This strong spirituality should not be confused with the behavioral component of church attendance that is religiosity. Practically none of these women attended church although they all spoke of being raised in the church. However, as the years went on church attendance was not seen as important. It is the spirituality, a cognitive process, that was enduring. This is an internal process of thinking about one's relationship to God or a higher being, to others, and to the world, which is experienced as prayer. It is a process that evolves throughout life.

## Community Mothers

In the African American community there are women who will mother young people who are not their biological children (Sparks, 1996). It is a caring response that is not tied to biological reproduction. These women play an important protective and socialization role in poor communities. They are role models for younger people, giving guidance and help in time of need. They are nurturing women who place themselves in relation to others. For those women whose HIV status was known in their communities, they did not feel stigmatized in their community mother role. Their voices tell the stories:

"I try to help the children in the building. If they need a quarter or 50 cents or whatever, I'll try to help. Crossin' the street, if they too small, I'll take them to the store and bring them back. If they out at night, I go get them and make sure they in the house. We look out for the children. Certain people, not everybody in the building. When I get my food stamps I buy everybody ices or these 10-cent blow pops 'cause they're cheaper. . . . It's something small, but to them it's a big thing, 'cause a lot of parents don't have time."

Some of the women tried to talk to younger women about their sexual activity:

"I tried to talk to her. I even wanted to adopt the baby and because she was getting pregnant too often and her mother was giving her too many abortions. I said when she gets ready and she really wants children, she won't be able to 'cause you can't keep tearing the body down and think it's gonna keep reproducing. Gotta preserve your body."

Messages about risky sexual behavior were also given:

"I have my little HIV books, and I coming through the street. I tell them to get tested, and they take my advice. I be givin' out pamphlets. I say, 'You better stop drugs 'cause you're hurtin' yourself.' Now they're gettin' busted, and the streets are gettin' clean. One girl came and asked me, and I brought her to the clinic."

Another woman on the same subject:

"I talked to her about diseases, because I know her lifestyle. I talk to her about HIV, because she is promiscuous and I'm fearful and it's like . . . 'Oh, well, I know him. He's been in jail for about 2 years. Well, that's the reason why you should be thinking about using a condom.' "

These women are generating resistance as they live their daily lives. They are strategic in these acts of community mothering, but do not see themselves as politically astute or brave. They show a resistance to having young people taken out of their communities by behaviors that place them in high-risk situations. This protection has historical significance in the African American communities where youth are in danger from forces inside and outside of the community.

## STRENGTH IN THE FACE OF ADVERSITY

The voices of the women give a picture of strength in the face of adversity. They value their children and grandchildren. They reach out to others. They do not focus on themselves. They resist oppressive conditions and cope actively with their illness and the daily challenges of life. They resist the stigma placed on them by others and use themselves in strategic ways to help others. This behavior is culturally congruent with cultural norms of African Americans in which the group is valued above the individual.

They know they are ill and may die, yet they do not focus on themselves as pitiful. The focus on the self is in service to their families and communities. It is seen in the themes that describe how stigma is viewed, how relationships with children and their own mothers are negotiated, how spirituality is embraced, and the community is engaged. The mother–daughter relationship for some is an open relationship of mutual empathy and emotional connectedness; for others it is a strained relationship with emotional tension. Sons are not as problematic, although it is not clear from the information I gathered why this is so. Many women do not tell of their HIV-positive diagnosis because they fear rejection from their close relatives. They suffer guilt and shame in doing this, but they also want to stay connected to their families. Although I did not ask directly about what had happened in the relationships, my clinical sense was that these HIV-positive mothers had been experienced by their daughters as abandoning and not protective, especially if the mothers had been involved in drugs. Additionally, the mothers of the HIV-positive women I interviewed may have viewed their daughters' behavior as painful, and thus an emotional distance developed. The interesting question is whether these women's illness will be a critical event that will forge a new relationship in the three-generation mother–daughter bond. My experience is that all of these women will have bouts of serious illness, even though new drugs have prolonged life for some. When illness becomes a reality, will the roles reverse as the daughter reaches out to the mother and perhaps becomes the caretaker?

These women are marginalized in ways that middle-class women cannot imagine. I marvel at their lack of anger. They are resistant to the socially constructed notions of who they are because of where they have come from. They do not focus on themselves. They help us understand that their lives are more than about "me"; they are about families and community. Their spirituality helps them be resistant to the forces of the illness and their life circumstances. We have much to learn from their stories.

## *ACKNOWLEDGMENTS*

I wish to thank Drs. Mary Jane Rotheram-Borus, Robert Bayer, Robert Klitzman; Mrs. Maryse Joseph; and the HIV Center for Clinical and Behavioral Studies, New York State Psychiatric Institute, Columbia University. This research was made possible by a grant from Brown University and a minority faculty grant supplement to Grant No. NIMH 499855.03 (Principal Investigator, Mary Jane Rotheram-Borus, Department of Psychiatry, UCLA).

## REFERENCES

Arimstead, L., & Forehead, R. (1995). For whom the bell tolls: Parenting decisions and challenges faced by mothers who are HIV positive. *Clinical Psychology: Science and Practice, 2,* 239–250.

Auerbach, J. D., Wypijewska, C., & Brodie, H. (Eds.). (1994). *AIDS and behavior: An integrated approach.* Washington, DC: National Academy Press.

Centers for Disease Control and Prevention. (1996). US AIDS cases reported through December, 1995. *HIV/AIDS Surveillance Report, 7,* 1–39.

Centers for Disease Control and Prevention. (1997). US AIDS cases reported through December, 1996. *HIV/AIDS Surveillance Report, 8,* 24–40.

Dorn, N., Henderson, S., & South, N. (Eds.). (1994). *AIDS: Women, drugs and social care.* London: Falmer Press.

Haverkos, H. W., & Quinn, T. C. (1995). The third wave: HIV infection among heterosexuals in the US and Europe. *International Journal of STD and AIDS, 6,* 227–232.

Hirschhorn, L. (1995). *AIDS Reader, 5,* 99–105.

Ickovics, J. R., & Rodin, J. (1992). Women and AIDS in the United States: Epidemiology, natural history, and mediating mechanisms. *Health Psychology, 11*(1), 1–16.

Kurth, A. (1993). *Until the cure.* New Haven, CT: Yale University Press.

Maslanka, H., Lee, J., & Freudenberg, N. (1995). An evaluation of community-based HIV services for women in New York State. *Journal of the American Medical Association, 3–4,* 121–126.

Ogbu, J. (1988). Class stratification, racial stratification and schooling. In L. Weiss (Ed.), *Class, race and gender in American education.* Albany, NY: State University of New York Press.

Schiller, N. (1993). The invisible women: Caregiving and the construction of AIDS health services. *Culture, Medicine and Psychiatry, 17,* 487–512.

Sherr, L., Hawkins, C., & Bennett, L. (1996). *AIDS as a gender issue: Psychosocial perspectives.* London: Taylor & Francis.

Smith, A., & Stewart, A. J. (1983). Approaches to studying racism and sexism in Black women's lives. *Journal of Social Issues, 39,* 1–15.

Sparks, E. (1996). Overcoming stereotypes of mothers in the African American context. In K. F. Wyche & F. Crosby (Eds.), *Women's ethnicities: Journeys through psychology.* Boulder, CO: Westview Press.

Wyche, K. F. (1993). Psychology and African American women: Findings from applied research. *Applied and Preventive Psychology, 2,* 115–121.

Wyche, K. F., & Lobato, D. (1996). Minority mothers: Stress and coping when your child is in special education. In K. F. Wyche & F. Crosby (Eds.), *Women's ethnicities: Journeys through psychology.* Boulder, CO: Westview Press.

# Conversation Two

Edited by

## KATHY WEINGARTEN

DESPITE the arbitrary arrangement of the chapters, several themes emerged in Conversation One. Among them were the centrality of loss and isolation in these mothers' experiences as well as blame and self-blame. Across the first four chapters we could see the oppressive effects of the Western constructs of individualism, self-sufficiency, and the narrowly defined family. These mothers interact with multiple systems, each of which significantly affects their lives for either good or ill. We saw in the first conversation that resistance can take the form of creating and sustaining mutual connections. The themes of both marginalization and resistance are touched on in the following conversation, and other themes begin to emerge as well.

CYNTHIA GARCÍA COLL: Both single mothers and lesbian mothers challenge the norm of heterosexual nuclear families.

PHOEBE KAZDIN SCHNITZER: That is an important issue to put on the table. This is not about mothers only but families themselves. Nontraditional configurations are occurring at this time and this begs for acknowledgment. Many nontraditional family structures exist, and not just families headed by single moms or lesbian or gay couple.

CYNTHIA GARCÍA COLL: It isn't even only about family structure. The presence of a man in a particular family doesn't make that family "right," "wrong". When we focus on structure, we miss the point that families are also about processes.

JANET L. SURREY: In Western cultures, the dominant family structure is patriarchal, with the father at the center. When we look at function, the idea of family shifts so that we pay attention to the relationships among those who are present.

LAURA BENKOV: For instance, donor insemination is a major threat to the patriarchal family structure. Donor insemination used to be reserved for married couples, and the message was very clear: They were the "real" families. These messages from the outside get into our psyches; the outside becomes inside. My daughter spends a lot of time sorting out the world without negatives or positives attached to the things she comes across. "I have one mommy; my friend has two mommies." She is sorting out the world very matter of factly, without judgment. However, the time for this kind of nonevaluative thinking is short. The culture's negative and positive judgments are powerful stuff.

JANET L. SURREY: My 5-year-old daughter is designing her fantasy family. She thinks two moms and a dad is a great idea. (*We all laugh and agree with her.*)

LAURA BENKOV: I felt a huge connection to Bonnie Ohye's work. It is a very particular way of speaking about biculturalism. It makes vivid her sense of the difficulty in keeping a balance between honoring Japanese culture while also honoring her daughters' different experiences with it. I think it is an extremely hard line to walk. Right now, my daughter's big thing is Cinderella and weddings and "someday my prince will come." So I'm having to think about how I can talk to her about these stereotypically hetereosexist images and also let her be herself.

BONNIE Y. OHYE: Those moments are difficult. We think things exist "out there" but find they have come into our families anyway. I think that happens to all the mothers in this book. In my case, I only have to look at my biracial daughters and see their physical similarities and differences to be reminded that they are the same, but also different from me. It must be more difficult when a mother does not have a constant reminder.

CYNTHIA GARCÍA COLL: In Bonnie Ohye's chapter, there is also a sense of loss. The context is not the one that is familiar to her, that shaped her. I am raising kids who are tricultural. Unlike me, they will never be wholly Puerto Rican; that will never be part of their experience. There is an incredible sense of loss—of struggling with who they are, with how I would like them to be, and with how the world asks them to be.

KATHY WEINGARTEN: For lesbian and single mothers and mothers who live in bicultural families, there is not just a sense of straddling two worlds, but of embodying two worlds. The mothers with HIV and AIDS, are also living in two worlds, the world of the "well" and, at times, that of the "dying."

JANET L. SURREY: In terms of resistance, there is something significant about children entering a different world from the one their mothers experience. The quality that mothers want to encourage is the capacity for resistance. This is apparent with all the mothers. How do you help children develop and keep that capacity?

LAURA BENKOV: With regard to being a single mom, there are definitely some advantages. Yet we don't hear about that. I put a gate up to protect myself from the negative messages. I think I make different choices at different times about filtering them out. But there are times that I don't necessarily want to put a gate up; I want to honor differences. I want to say to my children, "This difference—whatever it may be—is fine. You can be this."

CYNTHIA GARCÍA COLL: Is that the mother's perspective for the child? How will the child feel, because kids, to a certain extent, don't want to be different?

PHOEBE KAZDIN SCHNITZER: But it is important how mothers tell the story of their families, because the narratives mothers tell, the ones that address the differences in their families, are potential sites of resistance.

CYNTHIA GARCÍA COLL: I find a parallel between Karen Wyche's chapter on mothers with HIV/AIDS and Bonnie Ohye's chapter on biculturalism, a theme of collectivism versus individualism. In both chapters there is an emphasis on thinking collectively. In Karen's, particularly, it is in terms of women adopting a sense of community and the ways that this influences their mothering experience.

BONNIE Y. OHYE: I had an emotional response to Karen Wyche's chapter. Part of me envies these women with HIV and AIDS—the way the community is set up to be un-self-conscious about being collective. It's hard to accept that I cannot take collectivism for granted as they seem to. When the value of "collective" is more an integral part of community, it is easier. I felt some wistfulness— how wonderful to rely on that community and take it for granted.

LAURA BENKOV: It is ironic that Bonnie speaks this way about the value of collectiveness. She is the carrier of collectivity, but she is alone with this in her social context. Now, to turn to a different aspect of this, one regarding the clinical discourse, it made me think about Phoebe Kazdin Schnitzer's vignettes about single mothers and the "knee Jerk" remarks that were made by clinicians during the case conferences.

PHOEBE KAZDIN SCHNITZER: For some of the single moms, the idea "he needs his father" is an idea that they themselves hold. One single mother I recall was so despairing about this that she was convinced she could not parent on her own. Society's devaluation and pessimism about single mothering is internalized and experienced by the single parents themselves.

KATHY WEINGARTEN: I think that you are talking about a mechanism by which things are stigmatized. A phrase like "he needs his father" is a conceptual shortcut. It globally describes a situation instead of looking at what is going on for a particular family. The phrase is catchy, like velcro; it sticks. But, it has no subtlety. However, even though a phrase may evoke a particular belief system, it is nevertheless a rough approximation of that belief system.

LAURA BENKOV: There is clinical rhetoric around the idea that a child needs his father. It is so much a part of the culture that it is difficult to see that rhetoric for what it is.

KATHY WEINGARTEN: Precisely. Because it saturates the culture, it convinces mothers who are single that they are doing something wrong, that *they* are wrong. Having this belief system embedded in culture highjacks lived experience.

PHOEBE KAZDIN SCHNITZER: Yes, prejudice always masks diversity.

KATHY WEINGARTEN: There is a loss in terms of the complexity and richness of who these mothers are.

JANET L. SURREY: Yes, and a loss in terms of the resources they are and can be to their children.

PHOEBE KAZDIN SCHNITZER: This is marginalization up close—moving from stereotypes to inhibited interactions.

# 9

## "Real" Mothers

### Adoptive Mothers Resisting Marginalization and Re-Creating Motherhood

BETSY SMITH

JANET L. SURREY

MARY WATKINS

"Are you her 'mother'?"
"Is she yours?"
"Does she call you 'Mom'?"
"She can't be your baby. Where does she come
    from?"
"How much did she cost?"
    —*Comments directed to the authors by strangers at
    playgrounds, restaurants, and supermarkets*

T HE paths to and through motherhood differ in significant ways for adoptive and nonadoptive mothers. Some come to adoption through the disappointments of infertility, secretly harboring a sense that adoption is "second best." Others may choose adoption for personal, political, or moral reasons, despite voices that warn them against the "bad seed," or the "dangers" of going beyond one's bloodline. Adoptive mothers-to-be, rather than fathers, are often in charge of painstakingly arranging the adoption, as though it were an analogue to carrying a child. The desire to mother must sustain itself, under intense scrutiny from strangers at social agencies, through the wait for an assigned child and the pain of a match that falls through. There is no word like miscarriage to mark and convey the loss of a child whose image has been carried in the mother's heart.

When new biological mothers seek out resemblances between their family and the child and share stories of deliveries and nursing, adoptive mothers are often left out. Their experiences of coming to and beginning mothering are not widely known, shared, or acknowledged. Thankfully, among adoptive mothers, there is conversation, particularly about the positive experiences, the "birth stories" of adoption, of feeling called to mother a particular child, of a profound opening to what is initially "other," of the joy of seeing and holding their child for the first time, of the memory of the first moment the child feels like "one's own," and of the deep physical and psychological connection with one's child that feels fundamentally different from that with other children. We, the authors, know these joys personally because we are all adoptive mothers.

We also know of the more frightening and worrisome thoughts of adoptive mothers in mainstream North American culture. Twisted around our own and others' experiences of mothering, there is a legacy of cultural hesitation and apprehension about adoptive motherhood, based on dominant European American beliefs about the primacy of blood ties,[1] ethnocentricity, and traditional patriarchal inheritance systems. These beliefs live too in our psyches and place a burden of doubts, prescriptions, and responsibilities on us as adoptive mothers, which separate us from biological ones.

Thoughts like the following are familiar to us and to many adoptive mothers—indeed they have haunted us, but they are rarely spoken about. Although most mothers phrase their doubts in very personal terms, questions like those below can be traced back to cultural beliefs and ideologies, and the psychological models that reflect them. When traced to their roots, these thoughts can then be illumined, articulated, wrestled with, and challenged.

"Will my baby's attachment and love be as deep, strong, and resilient as a biological child's?"

"Will I be less attached to my child, and she or he to me, because we did not have the experiences of childbearing, nursing, or being together directly after birth?"

[1]This has been named "biologism" by Elizabeth Bartholet (1993, p. 93).

"Can my nurturing compensate for the often multiple losses my adoptive child has suffered: losses of birthparents, birth siblings, extended birth family, sometimes of birth country and culture?"

"Will differences in appearance make us seem less like a family?"

"Will these differences make my child feel uncomfortable and cause her to separate from me . . . and possibly from her siblings?"

"Will I, a white parent, fail to teach my child of color how to protect herself or himself in a racist culture?"

"Will my child ultimately leave me to join her or his kind?"

"Can nurture make up for being the product of a rape, being abandoned, having a biological mother or father who used drugs or alcohol or smoked?"

"Will I feel ill equipped at preparing and protecting my child as she or he navigates through what may be frightening and unfamiliar territory to me?"

"If I hold an optimistic or hopeful view, am I in serious denial regarding the wounds of adoption that will eventually hurt my child?"

We, the authors, are writing from our own experience, and we hope also to reflect the voices of many other adoptive mothers. Although some of our understanding comes from our personal stories, some also is from the stories of adoptive mothers we have witnessed in psychotherapy, in friendship, and in research (Watkins & Fisher, 1993). We are all white, relatively privileged women who have adopted internationally, and thus we are not representative of a vast number of adoptive families in this country. We are aware of the wealth of experience, strength, and cultural resources of adoptive mothers further outside the dominant culture. For example, adoption in African American culture has a profoundly different history, meaning, and value based on the ideal of collective responsibility for children. This grew out of the forced destruction of nuclear family relationships during slavery as well as from a far stronger sense of collective identity and the presence of extended family networks within African American families. Similarly, within Latino cultures, adoption of young children within and across families is a frequent occurrence, reflected in the familiar term *madre de crianza* or "childrearing mother."

Our children, adopted internationally, represent about 9%

(11,000) of the 127,000 adoptions legally recorded in the United States (Lewin, 1997). Our personal experiences do not speak directly to some of the contemporary American experiences of open domestic adoptions, to controversies surrounding African American adoptions into European American families, or to the issue of access to records to search for birth mothers.

I, Mary Watkins, came to adoption from a childhood of imagining a large family of adopted children. I began by being a stepparent to three. From that experience, I learned I could love a child who wasn't seen as "mine." From working with children clinically and being attuned to the international situation regarding children who need families, I found I could make better meaning out of adopting children than "having my own." I live in a multicultural, multiracial family with my husband and three daughters from Brazil, India, and China. It was through my study of motherhood cross-culturally and cross-historically that I first began to see clearly the use of psychological theory to promote dominant cultural ideologies, which then affect mothers' daily experience. It is my hope that mothers can collaboratively and intentionally create structures of mothering that support their children's and their own development. Despite the difficulties of adoptive family life, I am deeply moved by the reality and vision of love and nurture moving beyond the borders of blood, race, and ethnicity.

I, Betsy Smith, am an adoptive mother of two young children who were born in China. My female partner and I are jointly raising our children. I chose adoption after years of experiencing infertility and having been entrenched in the belief that a biologically related child would be the best choice, the most likely way of feeling the deepest sense of closeness with a child as well as somehow being easiest for my children. I have grown immeasurably in 6 years and have opened my heart and mind to the new ways I now envision and experience my own family. Becoming a biracial, bicultural family has been filled with challenges and surprises that my partner and I have tried to embrace fully. Both of us bring to our family the experience of living as lesbians in this culture, which I feel enables us to give our children a perspective on being outside the mainstream. Developing a positive self-image as a lesbian in a homophobic society involves a parallel "resistance" to the dominant cultural messages that pervade our world. I hope this perspective becomes a strength I can give my children over time.

I, Janet L. Surrey, am a Jewish, Buddhist, married, adoptive mother of Katie, my 6-year-old daughter born in China. My decision to adopt after a short period of infertility was partially a resistance to any further expensive and intrusive medical treatment. The decision to adopt has allowed me to reconnect to an early childhood dream ("I want to provide a home to a child who really needs one") as well as to an adolescent political statement ("The world is too endangered and overpopulated to give birth to more children"). Since Katie's arrival at 4 months old, I have been learning about the intersections of adoption, race, class, and gender status as these construct the adoption experience in this culture. At the same time, I hold a spiritual vision of adoption as a pathway toward the creation of a "global human family" and the most powerful commitment to diversity and multiculturalism I can live. I am obsessed daily with how to help Katie decode and challenge the messages she receives about her adoptive and racial status as well as with my responsibility to help create a world that will see, hear, value, and support her in her journey.

## THE CULTURAL CONSTRUCTION OF ADOPTION

The experiences of adoptive mothers challenge some of the most basic Western assumptions about what is "right," "normal," "real," "natural," and psychologically sound in family life. These assumptions are so strong that it comes as a surprise to find that in nature itself, among animals, adoption is quite common, both within and between species (Masson & McCarthy, 1995).

Adoption is as old as recorded history. Whether or not adoption is considered "normal" varies widely within different cultures, as does whether or not a culture grants equivalent kinship, legal, and inheritance status. Adoption often has been seen as a legitimate means of building families, resolving conflicts between families, ensuring inheritance and security in old age, and providing a "better" life for children (Bartholet, 1993). Ideas about adoption, then, must always be viewed as embedded within a particular cultural and historical context.

In North America, adoption has been constructed and understood within prevailing psychological models of human development that are also reflective of underlying cultural beliefs. These models support the idea that adoption places children at risk. Most research on adoption in the United States has focused on "outcome" studies, where the success of adoption has been studied with emphasis placed on exploring psychological risk factors (Brodzinsky & Schecter, 1990). The belief is widespread that adoptees have more psychological problems than nonadoptive peers. Only recently has it been suggested that rates of referral of adoptive children to mental health facilities may be affected by cultural beliefs. Warren (1992) suggested that the status of adoption itself significantly increases the likelihood of referral for psychiatric treatment of adolescents. Adoptees are significantly more likely to be referred even when they display fewer problems than nonadoptees. The author concluded that overrepresentation of adoptees in clinical settings is not attributable solely to the fact that they may be more troubled, but to cultural beliefs that expect them to be so. Over the past century, until quite recently, much of the writing and psychological reflection on adoption has undermined the confidence and optimism of adoptive mothers. Very little attention has been paid to the actual lived experience and the enormous care, courage, personal commitment, and growth so often involved in such parenting.

We suggest in this chapter that we need to study the sources of psychological strength and developmental pathways that lead to healthy resistance in adoptive families in general and in mothers in particular. Adoptive mothering offers unique challenges, opportunities for growth, and experiences of risk and adventure in the embracing of diversity and the creation of family relationships, typically without personal or familial models.

The impact of adoption on mothers' development is clearly very powerful. New work has begun to detail the relational practice of adoptive mothering (Watkins & Fisher, 1993), to make available the stories of adoptive mothers, adoptive daughters, and birth mothers (Wadia-Ells, 1995), and to give voice to white adoptive mothers' experience and learning about racism (Lazarre, 1996; Reddy, 1996).

We believe that one of the greatest sources of resistance and empowerment for adoptive mothers is the recognition and analysis of the power of cultural marginalization and psychological pathologizing of their experience and that of their children. To see this power one can look at how adoption is and is not represented in the arts, media, film, schools, and mental health systems. For example, we can examine the sensational highlighting of tearful "reunion" stories between children and birth mothers in the media, or the lack of representation of adoption in books for children or in elementary school curriculum on families.[2] The degree to which adoption is pathologized is still seen in

[2]One of the authors wrote a children's book on adoption, which was rejected by publishers, who said it would be of interest to only a very small percentage of the population.

issues of confidentiality around adoption in schools and the shaming of adopted children by peers.

Adoptive mothers struggle with their internalizations of cultural objections and ambivalence to the differences adoptive family life poses. They are often marginalized by nonadoptive mothers, as well as by society at large. In addition, they are caught, often unaware, in a cross-fire within the adoption community. In one camp are those who are ideologically committed to the idea that adoption as it is commonly practiced is a disservice to children, a breeding ground for almost inevitable psychopathology and identity disturbances. Phrases such as "primal wound," "genetic ego," and "genealogical bewilderment" abound in the literature. This side can be heard in the mass media and professional literature throughout the land. For example, a letter to the editor of *The Boston Globe* (Waldron, 1993) states a widely held opinion in this partial quote: "Until we truly understand that adoption is a profoundly unnatural act from which there is never full recovery, and that other choices must prevail . . . " The writer simply assumes this statement to be true, and goes on to make her next point without any hesitation.

In the other camp are those who believe that adoption can be a positive experience for children, that it is the manner in which the differences of adoption are addressed that determines the outcome. Indeed, the latter argues that recovery from the losses of adoption within the supportive intimacy of a good-enough adoptive home may well contribute to a more robust resiliency than is usually available to nonadopted peers (Drew, 1996).

We argue here that the mental health and psychological development of adoptive mothers is, in part, dependent on coming to understand how cultural ideologies about adoption influence our thoughts and actions. Once this is recognized, adoptive mothers can draw on personal and collective power to challenge prevailing beliefs and to develop and "hold" an alternative belief system. In fact this process is at the heart of many "successful" adoptive parenting experiences. We are suggesting that this process can be more consciously articulated and supported by adoption communities and agencies; extended families and friends of adoptive families; mental health professionals; and educational, legal, and governmental institutions and policy makers, and through the responsible use of media. Adoptive mothers need to have clarity about the ideologies framing their experiences in order to approach them from an empowered position of challenging and transforming these ideas of motherhood and kinship in the light of their actual experience with their children. Without such a process, adoptive mothers remain on the margin, their experiences lost in reimagining motherhood and kinship.

## DOMINANT CULTURAL IDEOLOGIES AND BELIEFS

What do families that are marginalized because of their difference from the norm have to teach about motherhood? Our belief is that penetrating the forms of motherhood that seem "other" reveals something about those forms as well as about the dominant ideologies of our culture. Our hope is that by looking more closely at adoptive motherhood we can use it as a window through which we can see more clearly the largely unconscious but dominant ideologies of the family, the child, and motherhood. As Kirk (1964) and Wegar (1997) have eloquently pointed out, these ideologies largely concern issues of "difference" and the possibilities of relating across difference. Presently these issues around difference are as central to the evolution of our national and global identities as they are to the integrity of adoptive family life. In the end we shall learn some lessons from the metabolizing of differences within adoptive families; these lessons have the potential to speak to the problems of the larger culture.

Below we discuss the dominant ideologies that enshadow adoptive motherhood.

1. *The primacy and superiority of sameness; thus the valuing of blood relations over all others and the valuing of racial and cultural sameness.*

When similarity between child and parent is highly valued, blood children are sought, often regardless of pain and price for parents with fertility difficulties. Many infertile couples who truly wish to parent remain childless in order to avoid the uncertainties of harboring in their homes "the other," the genetically dissimilar.

Similarity between parents and child appears to be thought a virtue, even in cases when it flies in the face of rationality. For instance, a couple resists adopting a child because of the unknown difference in gene pool, even though a serious genetic disorder is known to exist in their own family lines. Additionally, same genes do not necessarily result in sameness. Often biological offspring look quite different from at least one parent depending on how the genes mix together. More subtle unexpected differences exist, too, among biologically related mothers and children, based on temperament and constitution.

Spanning both the dominant and African American cultures is a common assumption, although for different reasons, that children fare better when they are brought up in families that resemble them racially. Institutional racism is clearly evident in the enormous demand for "healthy, white infants" in preadoptive families, especially those who most closely "fit" the dominant culture's definition of the healthy "norm." The assumption that racial sameness yields better adoptive outcomes is contradicted by much research (Gill & Jackson, 1983; Figelman & Silverman, 1983); nonetheless, adoptive parents in transracial families are often marginalized by white families as well as by families of color. In addition, transracial families suffer under the prejudice within the adoption system that makes the adoption of black children by white parents particularly difficult, at times impossible. The National Association of Black Social Workers has worried, with good reason, that the adoption of black children into white families will leave these children unprepared and undefended against the massive assault of racism they will encounter in American society. Transracial adoptive mothers may well have to learn to confront and challenge both racism and "biologism" as powerful forces impacting them and their children. Recent writing suggests that white adoptive mothers may have a unique perspective to offer as they learn to negotiate for their children within biracial and multicultural contexts (Lazarre, 1996; Reddy 1996).

There are ways in which, by challenging the biological paradigm of building families, the adoptive mother's perspective on parenting yields insights into how families are constructed in our culture. Do the losses inherent for adoptive children and mothers necessitate tragedy? Or can they help to enrich the formation of a family that comes together with an initial effort that requires a belief that differences can be positive, that biological connections are not the only "real" ones that build families? Can there be a way that adoptive mothers can offer their children more opportunities to develop without the burden of expectations that sometimes weigh on biological children? Is there a way, particularly in cross-racial adoptive families, in which children may become better equipped for the increasingly multicultural world they are being raised in? Is there an opportunity for both mother and child to be more aware of, and allied with, other people who do not fit into mainstream images of family (single mothers, lesbian mothers, families with a special-needs child, etc.)?

2. *The developmental primacy of environmental nurture over genetic endowment.*

Paradoxically, another cultural ideology that has affected adoptive parents—although it is not as deep or as embedded—is exactly the opposite of this: Namely, biological inheritance is far less important in how children turn out than is the day-to-day environment in which they partake. The democracy of America is deeply influenced by the thinking of John Locke and the ideology of individualism that issued from it (Kagan, 1994). In order to break free of inherited rank, to have a culture in which, with the proper education, all citizens could inform their government and avail themselves of opportunity, it was necessary to minimize the importance of genetic endowment and emphasize the importance of environment. Wegar (1997) points out that this is a principal reason for adoption taking hold sooner in America than it did in England.

Further, after the atrocities of racism and anti-Semitism in the first half of our century, psychological research silenced study of racial differences for several decades after World War II (Kagan, 1994). During this time, which coincided with the ascendancy of adoption, nurture was further lauded in the field of psychology for its effects over nature.

History fuels these contradictory messages about adoption. The predominant belief in the 1950s and 1960s was that adoption was the "perfect solution" to illegitimacy and infertility among white women.[3] However, in the 1970s, critics of adoption claimed that adoption created a rupture of biological kinship that could be harmful for parents and children (Melosh, 1994).

Given the strength of cultural commitment to the value of sameness, the parallel, though opposite, belief in the importance of nurture placed adoption practice in an awkward position, which was

---

[3]There are two very different histories of single pregnancy in the post-World War II era: for black women and for white women. Both were shunned and humiliated by a variety of institutions because of their predicament, but white unmarried women who became pregnant were often "sent away" to relatives or homes to complete the pregnancy and then have the child adopted by people outside the family. This solution was possible because there was a growing pressure on white women to become mothers during the "baby boom" years after the war and the number of births among out-of-wedlock white women was rising. Black women, however, were told by social service agencies that their children were not adoptable, and relatives generally became the caretakers. Differing "value" was attached to children based on race, fueling the still present societal rage at illegitimate black children (see Solinger, 1992, for a detailed history of this issue).

reflected by some of the logical inconsistencies in adoption practice. For instance, families were reassured that nurture was the most important factor while babies were carefully matched with parents for appearance, religion, and social class. Further, adoption records were sealed, in part to prevent adoptive parents from being alarmed by the differences between themselves and the adopted child. However, purportedly this was done "in the best interests of the child," and it was proselytized that the history of the biological parents would have little bearing on the child's development, which was deemed to be affected primarily by the social bonds within the adoptive home. At worst, these contradictions complicate the adoption experience for all involved. It is remarkable, given the conflicting messages, that in fact many adoptive families live out a healthy and creative integration of these apparently opposing belief systems.

3. *The purported importance of "bonding" to the mother–child relationship.*

As if this contradiction weren't powerful enough, adoptive mothers since the 1970s have had to deal with the romanticization of the interaction between mother and child in the early hours after birth. Klaus and Kennell's (1976) work on mother–baby bonding, based on now-refuted ideas and research, claimed that a future of maternal child abuse and neglect would be more likely if a mother did not bond with her newborn in the first few hours of birth. They claimed that without this experience a mother was more likely to neglect or abuse her child, or fail to attach, in a way that would leave a hole in the psyche of the child (Eyer, 1992). Because most adoptive mothers adopt their children after this infamous "critical period," they are believed to be unable to inoculate their relationship with their baby from these dreadful outcomes. The theory of bonding, as Eyer (1992) beautifully educates us, is still used, despite its downfall in research and theory, because it supports underlying cultural beliefs. Mothers, he says, are not educated to differentiate between bonding and attachment, the latter describing the unfolding of a relational connection of trust and reliance over time. Giving birth, nursing, and being with the child directly after birth are not ingredients essential to the development of the mother's attachment to the child, or to the child's attachment to the mother.

The mother–infant bonding research is yet another example in which adoptive mothers basically can't be "real" mothers. "Real" relationships that will "hold" or "last" are based on biological "blood" ties and the immediate bonding supposedly made after birth. Relational connections based on love, empathy, mutuality, and commitment are not seen as strong enough, that is, they will not "hold" through time, geographic distance, conflict, or contact with biological kin.

Adoptive mothers are left struggling with the fear that they are not strong enough to provide the proper relational matrix. The relationship is somehow diminished and seen as being less sustaining, less potent, more fragile, and all in all less "real" than relationships based on "blood" and bonding at birth. There clearly is evidence that infants develop a sense of familiarity with their biological mother even prenatally, and there can be important effects of relationship disruption. However, these observations do not contradict the fact that adoptive mothers can, and usually do, learn to work with this, neither denying nor despairing about this fact.

4. *The psychological health of the child is dependent solely on the relationship with the "nuclear family" mother.*

This notion has become so ingrained in American psychology that it blinds us to our recent historical past and to the childcare arrangements of cultures other than in North America. Before industrialization, children were taken care of by a host of caretakers who included older siblings, apprentices living in the family, and extended family as well as parents. In white colonial America, as John Demos (1983) has shown, the outcome of a child's character was thought to be dependent on the father's influence, not the mother's.

Once fathers left home for the workplace, apprentices left also, and families became more nuclear (less extended kin living together). Childcare was then relegated to the mother. It is only at that time, a little over 100 years ago, that the relationship with the mother began to be thought of as significant, and then crucial, for the child's psychological development, especially as advanced by psychoanalytic theory (see Introduction).

Historically, in African American and Latino families there has been greater reliance on extended family for the raising of a child. Even in language, there is room made for both biological mothers and mothers who are not kin through blood, but through the daily care of the child: "blood mothers" and "othermothers" for African Americans (Hill-Collins, 1991), and *madres de sangre* (blood mothers) and *madres de crianza* (childrearing mothers) for Latinos. In many cultures, the "real," most valued mothers are not necessarily the biological ones, but rather the adult women who actually take on more of the parenting responsibilities. The increasing number of lesbian families in North America in which there are two mothers parenting children also challenges the notion of one primary mother in the construction of a family (Benkov, 1994). In these examples, the child can be seen to profit from a collaboration among caretakers. Multiplicity of mothering figures is not seen negatively, as it is seen in contemporary Eurocentric psychological models.

The analogous situation in adoptive family life is clear: birth mothers and adoptive mothers, and sometimes foster mothers and orphanage mothers on the way to the adoptive home. This multiplicity has been seen exclusively through the lens of loss, given our monocular view of child development being reliant on the child's relation with a single caretaker. Looking cross-culturally and historically this view needs to be supplemented by a vision of the child as being cared for by a nexus of adults, which can include birth and adoptive families, fathers and mothers, siblings and extended family, and institutions, including schools and religious communities as well as orphanages and foster families.

However, in a culture that values blood relations over others, the parents considered "real" are the birth parents, despite any acts they have committed that are antithetical to "parenting." Young children, unschooled in the biology of genetics, learn this early on. It is not unusual for an adoptive child of 6 to speak about her or his birthparents as "real," and the adoptive parents as "not real." This dichotomizing— real–unreal—is an extension of our limiting in language and reality the number of caretakers of our children, clearly giving priority to blood.

Birth mothers and adoptive mothers are too often depicted as in competition, and their relationship is defined as "winning" or "losing" (Melosh, 1994). The cultural paradigm attempts to dictate that they be divided, separated, in conflict, and mutually threatening. Adoptive mothers fear that birth mothers will "claim" their children, legally or psychologically. Birth mothers feel cast out or vilified by society in general and often by adoptive mothers. The media plays on this by highlighting stories of highly emotional reunions of children and birth mothers and wrenching custody battles between adoptive and birth mothers.

The open adoption movement has attempted to address this unnecessary division and support all the relationships within the adoption triangle (child, birth parent, and adoptive parent), but often underlying fears and perceived threats may still impact the unfolding relationships. These adoptions do not yet take place in a culture that supports multiplicity of mothering and solidarity among mothers.

However, many successful experiments in open adoption today *are* challenging these assumptions of division and competition among mothers.

Revisioning the relationship between mothers as mutually enhancing, supportive, and grounded in responsibility for children, both in the adoption triangle and in the culture at large, would profoundly reshape the configuration and context of adoption. We believe this ideology of basic conflict and mutual threat is an enormous source of difficulty for both adoptive and birth mothers. Conversely, the revisioning of this relationship by adoptive mothers, birth mothers, and their children can be an enormous contribution to the task of resisting and reframing such cultural ideologies. Collaborative parenting based on empathic care for children rather than notions of ownership support the psychological development of parents as well as children.

## 5. *An identity that is simple is superior to one that is complex.*

One fallout from the cultural derogation of difference is a cultural premise that it is better for a child to have a simple identity than a complex one. When one adds the differences of race and culture to that of adoption itself, this premise argues that adopted children will have identity confusion that will weaken their sense of self. Elsewhere, Watkins and Fisher (1993) have argued that the fact that children must knit together the various pieces of a complex identity neither means that they will fail this task nor that this task handicaps them in any way. On the contrary, it can be argued that work on this very task of a heterogeneous identity prepares these children in a unique way for participation in a multicultural society and world where the negotiation of difference is an essential skill.

Similarly, for adoptive mothers, messages from the dominant culture generally warn women that the task of becoming an adoptive mother may be difficult, confusing, and complicated, particularly if it is a cross-racial adoption. Rarely is there encouragement that the process could be expansive in terms of one's identity. If circumstances permit, however, there is the potential for exploring new parts of oneself in becoming an adoptive mother. There is often a parallel growth of mother and child as a mutual relationship develops that acknowledges and respects differences. When a white mother adopts a child of another race, the way she understands herself, the world, and the experiences of people of color begins to change. No longer is she able to see the world only as a white person without having a perception of how people view her and her child as somehow different. Antennae are up when discussions of race occur at work, when children at the playground question where the mother of her child is, when political events take place that are related to race and need to be explained to her child. There can be an internal strengthening that develops, an assertiveness that may be newly experienced as the woman rises to advocate for her child or to learn about the child's cultural heritage. Just as biracial or bicultural intimate relationships for adults can be a catalyst for change in how each person experiences her or his identity, multiracial families provide a parent with new opportunities for forging a more complex and multifaceted sense of self.

6. *Adoptive mothers are defective as mothers, causing psychiatric symptoms in their adopted children.*

Issuing from the work of psychoanalyst Helene Deutsch (1945) is the judgment that infertile adoptive mothers are unable to parent success-fully. This purportedly has to do with the narcissistic wound to them caused by their infertility, which may have originally been an uncon-scious rejection of motherhood. Infertility in this model is equated with feelings of inferiority in the psyche of the mother that so preoccupy her that she cannot give enough maternal love to her child. Schecter (1960) continues in this tradition warning that the adoptive child is a constant reminder to the mother of her "barrenness." These bleak prognostica-tions claim that such maternal issues result in increased psychiatric disorder among adoptees. They do not pause to consider that the stigmatizing itself places all members of the adoptive family at risk for psychological hardship (Kirk, 1964; Watkins & Fisher, 1993; Wegar, 1997). Clinical observations suggest that there are actually strengths as well as vulnerabilities associated with parenting after infertility (Glazer, 1990).

7. *Adoption is a lifelong grieving process for all members of the adoption triangle.*

Certainly there are losses and various periods of grieving related to the adoption experience that birth mothers, adoptive mothers, and adopted children face at different developmental points. Until recently the voices of many birth mothers had been silenced, with much of their grief having been endured quietly by themselves.

However, the seemingly relentless focus by clinicians on the perpetual grieving process for those directly affected by adoption is often what adoptive mothers confront when seeking support and guidance. When challenged with the notion that she will be unable to impact this grief substantially for her child, the adoptive mother is faced with an enormous sense of helplessness. Rarely is she counseled that adoption is as much recovery from loss as it is loss itself (Bernard, 1974). Feelings of anger, disappointment, and loss can often be directed between birth mother, adoptive mother, and adopted child, which can intensify the fears that each member of the triangle may hold. If, instead, all the voices of children, birth mothers, and adoptive mothers could be heard and better understood, then the grief might not be seen as an inevitable, ongoing psychological construction.

The adoptive mother is cast in the role of forestalling or beating the terrible odds she is given by the culture around her. She feels the pressure from numerous sources to be a better than ordinary mother in order to prove her entitlement to the child and to compensate for the "damages" already done as well as those considered to be endemic to living the adoptive life. This defensive posture makes it difficult to step away and clearly evaluate the forms of attack she is negotiating and to articulate the values her family and her mothering represent.

Further, because adoption is most often pursued because of infertility, not from choice, there is no reason to believe that adoptive mothers begin their journey with a conscious sensibility regarding the cultural norms by which they are entrapped. Indeed, they often begin, sadly enough, by thinking that adoption is second best, that adoptive children grow up flawed, that the love they will receive from an adoptive child is more fragile than that from a "natural" child, and that the love they must give may go beyond their capacities and still fail to fortify their children sufficiently. Disappointment about needing to adopt is shameful to admit openly and difficult to bear alone. How much the cultural ideas and psychological representations of these beliefs contribute to this disappointment! Adoptive mothers further along in their questioning of these ideas, and further along in their own experience of not only the challenges of adoptive motherhood, but the beauty and hope of it, have a critical role to play in creating a more positive cultural outlook on adoptive family life.

## SOURCES OF RESISTANCE

Cultural ideologies live and are either reproduced or challenged within our psyches and our actions. These ideas place a set of burdensome thoughts and responsibilities on the adoptive mother that haunt her silently, that are difficult for her to articulate and still more difficult to fight and transform. And yet the metabolization of this cultural residue is critical to her own mental health, to her relationship to her children, and to her ability to give voice and power to her own experience.

There are various arenas that both impact and are impacted by the development of healthy cultural resistance (Weingarten, 1995) by adoptive mothers. Communities—both the adoptive community and other communities to which families relate—are a source of support and, at times, a place for education by adoptive mothers. There are important lessons for the mental health and research worlds to learn from adoptive mothers. Clinicians, adoption workers, teachers, and health care providers can be most helpful by moving beyond notions of emotional "support" to a model of supporting mothers' ability to resist the marginalization and pathologizing of their maternal experience and practice.

We believe that deconstructing the underlying dominant ideologies that construct adoption in mainstream American culture will liberate new energies and new visions of mothering, family, and human connectedness. We hope it will liberate the voices, strengths, and resources of adoptive mothers who are further marginalized by differences such as race, class, ethnicity, sexual identity, and disability status. This process of cultural resistance needs to be simultaneously undertaken at the personal and societal levels. We see the availability of and access to communities of resistance as essential to the liberating process.

We have found helpful a model of resistance based on Robinson and Ward's (1991) description of the process of repudiation and affirmation as an act of resistance for African American girls. We believe this may reflect a mother's developmental process as well as a cultural evolution of resistance.

The first form, *resistance for survival,* is an adaptation that lies in being as invisible as possible and calling little attention to oneself. This is often seen in an adoptive mother who may minimize differences in her adoptive family . She may rarely speak openly about being in an adoptive family, may keep the adoption secret to her child or others in her life, and may feel so uncomfortable about adoption that she evades and abbreviates such discussion. Adoptive mothers were prescribed this strategy by many adoption "experts" until recently.

The second form of resistance, *resistance for equality,* seeks equality under the law, with equal rights and representation in all areas. For example, adoptive mothers might encourage teachers and administrators to include adoption as an equal and positive option in creating families when developing curriculum, literature, and classroom activities. Tax credits, inheritance laws, benefits to support adoption costs, adoption leave for parents, and medical insurance that fairly includes children adopted with preexisting conditions are further examples. Adoption can be viewed as a form of diversity, and it intersects with multiculturalism as this becomes integrated into new belief systems.

The last form of resistance described by Robinson and Ward (1991) is *resistance for liberation*. This form of resistance challenges oppressive or destructive cultural norms and seeks to offer new visions and voices to the culture. Moving beyond a vision of simply experiencing equality, resistance for liberation would involve a profound reconceptualization of many aspects of our lives. In this regard adoptive mothers offer much in helping all people consider the social construction of family, the concept of "ownership" of children, the dangers of mother blaming that occur for all kinds of mothers, and mythologies regarding blood ties. An example of this kind of change would be parents working with teachers of elementary schools to transform curriculum on families. Instead of asking children to draw or write about their "family tree" (a more traditional way of conceptualizing families that emphasizes the centrality of blood ties), teachers could consider using a circle with the child in the center and then including important people in the child's life in outlying circles. This may more accurately capture the fuller relational matrix of not only adopted children but many children with multiple webs of relationships in all kinds of family structures.

The developmental path for adoptive mothers that we are prescribing is a liberatory path, drawn in part from the work of Paulo Freire, the leader of Brazil's literacy movement. Freire describes liberation as coming about in two stages. In the first, called *conscientization*, members of a group become aware of the cultural ideologies that shape their day-to-day life (Freire, 1989). In the second, *annunciation*, the group envisions in a more ideal fashion how things could be structured for the good. Adoptive mothers must become aware of the ideologies they labor under. They must identify the thoughts and feelings to which these ideologies give rise. They must radically question these thoughts and feelings, eventually disidentifying from ones that are not supportive of their families—both children and adults—created through adoption. We believe that this work is best done within a community of adoptive mothers whose membership promotes sharing among veteran adoptive mothers and newer ones who are particularly vulnerable to the stresses and stigmas we have outlined above. Through creative dialogue in such communities, we believe that adoptive families can actually begin to see themselves as pioneers in consciously constructing forms of family that serve children and honor difference and that aid in liberating other kinds of mothers from oppressive ideologies.

In addition to community building, reconceptualizing psychological models of adoption also leads to a more liberatory way of considering adoptive mothers. The psychiatric literature and research has caused significant damage and pain for many of them throughout this century. Until recently, with rare exceptions, the literature and advice to adoptive mothers and their children was dominated with images of the "primal wound" on the child and the inadequate "bonding" of adoptive mothers to their children. Clinicians working with adoptive mothers may want to consider "prescribing" or helping to create consciousness-raising groups for them and assisting clients in accessing other peer supports and resources to help build communities of resistance. Research projects that look at nonclinical populations of adoptive mothers and adopted children should be explored in greater depth. Continued development and reinforcement of nonblaming, nonjudgmental language to describe members of the adoption triangle are important, for example, birth mother, biological mother; instead of "real" mother, "natural" mother, or "abandoning" mother; adopted child instead of orphan. Use of language, such as "primal wound," that presents adoption as an affliction needs to be curtailed as well.

With the development of strong community networks for adoptive mothers, pressure can be applied in the political and policy-making arenas regarding adoption legislation and decisions. If serious consideration were given to the perspectives of adoptive mothers and children, community responses might be stronger in response to insensitive or inaccurate images about adoption represented in many places from the media to school curriculums.

## CONCLUSION

Adoptive mothers have much in common with other marginalized mothers in the path to liberation. The notions that guide our understanding of the possibility of reconstructing motherhood and family do not arise from adoption alone. We stand with other mothers whose lives and mothering practices challenge traditional views of what constitutes healthy families and good mothers, and that move us toward embracing a more experiential and relational definition of mothering (see especially Benkov, Chapter 5, and Schnitzer, Chapter 7, this volume). We support the cross-fertilization between and among different groups of marginalized mothers, both as a support to recognizing and deconstructing sources of marginalization and in evolving strategies of resistance. We offer this chapter in an effort to develop such an enlarged community with other mothers.

## REFERENCES

Bartholet, E. (1993). *Family bonds: Adoption and the politics of parenting.* Boston: Houghton Mifflin.

Benkov, L. (1994). *Reinventing the family: The emerging story of lesbian and gay parents.* New York: Crown.

Bernard, V. W. (1974). Adoption. In S. Arieti (Ed.), *American handbook of psychiatry* (Vol. I). New York: Basic Books.

Brodzinsky, D. M., & Schecter, M. D. (1990). *The psychology of adoption.* New York: Oxford University Press.

Demos, J. (1983). The changing faces of fatherhood: A new exploration in family history. In F. Kessel & A. Siegel (Eds.), *The child and other cultural inventions.* New York: Praeger.

Deutsch, H. (1945). *Psychology of women.* New York: Grune & Stratton.

Drew, T. (1996, July). *The resiliency factor: Implications for theory, practice, and policy.* Paper presented at the Annual Foster Care and Adoption Conference, Albuquerque, NM.

Eyer, D. (1992). *Mother–infant bonding: A scientific fiction.* New Haven, CT: Yale University Press.

Figelman, W., & Silverman, A. R. (1985). *Chosen children.* New York: Praeger.

Freire, P. (1989). *Pedagogy of the oppressed.* New York: Continuum.

Gill, O., & Jackson, B. (1983). *Adoption and race: Black, Asian and mixed race children in white families.* New York: St. Martin's Press.

Glazer, E. (1990). *The long awaited story: A guide to parenting after infertility.* New York: Macmillan Press.

Hill-Collins, P. (1991). The meaning of motherhood in Black culture and Black mother–daughter relationships. In P. Bell-Scott, B. Guy Sheftall, J. Jones Royster, J. Sims-Wood, M. DeCosta-Willis, & L. P. Fultz (Eds.), *Double stitch: Black women write about mothers and daughters.* New York: HarperPerennial.

Kagan, J. (1994). *Galen's prophecy: Temperament in human nature.* New York: Basic Books.

Kirk, H. D. (1964). *Shared fate: A theory and method of adoption and mental health.* New York: Free Press.

Klaus, M., & Kennell, J. (1976). *Mother–infant bonding: The impact of early separation or loss on family development.* St. Louis, MO: Mosby.

Lazarre, J. (1996). *Beyond the whiteness of whiteness: Memoir of a white mother of black sons.* Durham, NC: Duke University Press.

Lewin, T. (1997, November 9). U.S. is divided on adoption, survey of attitudes asserts. *The New York Times*, p. 16.

Masson, J., & McCarthy, S. (1995). *When elephants weep.* New York: Delacorte.

Melosh, B. (1994, April). *Adoption autobiography and the construction of identity.* Paper presented at annual convention of the Organization of American Historians. Atlanta, GA.

Reddy, M. (1996). *Crossing the color line: Race, parenting, and culture.* New Brunswick, NJ: Rutgers University Press.

Robinson, T., & Ward, J. (1991). A belief in self far greater than anyone's disbelief: Cultivating resistance among African American female adolescents. In C. Gilligan, A. Rogers, & D. Tolman (Eds.), *Women, girls and psychotherapy: Reframing resistance.* Binghamton, NY: Haworth Press.

Schecter, M. D. (1960). Observation of adopted children. *Archives of General Psychiatry, 3,* 21–33.

Solinger, R. (1992). *Wake up little Susie: Single pregnancy and race before Roe v. Wade.* New York: Routledge.

Wadia-Ells, S. (Ed.). (1995). *The adoption reader: Birth mothers, adoptive mothers and adopted daughters tell their stories.* Seattle: Seal Press.

Waldron, J. (1993, August 11). [Letter to the editor]. *The Boston Globe,* p. 20.

Warren, S. B. (1992). Lower threshold for referral for psychiatric treatment for adopted adolescents. *Journal of the American Academy of Child and Adolescent Psychiatry, 31*(3), 512–517.

Watkins, M., & Fisher, S. (1993). *Talking with young children about adoption.* New Haven, CT: Yale University Press.

Wegar, K. (1997). *Adoption, identity and kinship.* New Haven, CT: Yale University Press.

Weingarten, K. (1995). *Cultural resistance: Challenging beliefs about men, women, and therapy.* Binghamton, NY: Haworth Press.

# 10

❧

# Against All Odds
## Resistance and Resilience
## in African American Welfare Mothers

### ELIZABETH SPARKS

*I AM* an African American woman who grew up in the 1950s with friends and relatives who received "aid"—the colloquial term for the Aid to Dependent Children program. It was later also commonly called "welfare." Many of the families of children who attended my elementary school received this assistance, and my aunt and cousins were recipients of the "commodity food" distributed to the poor each month under this program. As a college student during the 1970s, I read descriptions of welfare-dependent families in the popular press, but I did not recognize the individuals described in this material. My aunt and friends' mothers were not lazy, promiscuous women who had different values from the rest of society. They were respectable, church-going women who instructed their children to get a good education so they could get good jobs and not become dependent on welfare. When they were able to find jobs, these women worked as private maids in the households of white families or as beauticians working out of their own kitchens, often being paid very little for their work. They scrimped and saved so their children could go to college, and they found ingenious ways to feed and clothe their families.

As a social worker during the 1980s, I visited the homes of many mothers who received Aid to Families with Dependent Children

(AFDC) and generally found these women to be similar to the mothers I had known in childhood. They struggled to keep homes that were orderly and clean. They also wanted the best for their children and hoped (and prayed) that they would escape from poverty and dependence on welfare. During the years when I was a protective services social worker, I also saw my share of welfare-dependent mothers who were drug addicted, neglectful, and abusive to their children. But they were the exception, not the rule. So, why weren't these hard-working women who were struggling against the odds presented in the popular media?

The voices and experiences of African American mothers were not found in this material nor were they the subject of academic discourse because of their marginalization within mainstream American culture. Marginalization is not a new phenomenon for African Americans. Our lives have been marginalized for over 200 years. During the era of slavery, African American women were considered "breeders" by slave masters, and their mothering was restricted to conception and birth (Greene, 1994). Infants could be, and often were, removed within a few months of birth, and even those who were allowed to remain with their mothers were generally taken care of by others during the long hours that their mothers worked in the fields. The end of slavery, however, did not bring about a corresponding end to the marginalization of African American mothers. Throughout our history in this country, African American women have had to confront such negative stereotypes as "Mammy," who is an asexual maternal figure caring for her white charges with self-sacrificial nurturance and devotion, and "Jezebel," who is an unfit mother because of her sexual promiscuity (Collins, 1990; Greene, 1994; Gilkes, 1994; Sparks, 1996).

The most recent stereotype, that of the "welfare mother," characterizes African American mothers on welfare as lazy, promiscuous women who are unable to adequately socialize their children. They are portrayed as "bad" mothers who do not provide an appropriate role model for their children because of their unemployment. They are blamed for their own poverty and are thought to need motivation to work, either through incentives or punishments (Fraser & Gordon, 1991). This characterization of low-income African American women serves to render their ideas, feelings, and mothering practices invisible and silent. They are forced out to the margins of society. Why are there such negative images of African American welfare mothers in the majority culture? This chapter represents my efforts to find an answer.

I have incorporated into the chapter the voices of four African American women who have received welfare at some point in their lives.[1]

Carla was a 34-year-old single woman who was currently attending a state university. She had two children (ages 7 and 12) and was hoping to enter a career where she could make an income that would allow her to care adequately for herself and her children in the future. Carla had both worked and received welfare in the past; she was currently a recipient while she completed her college education. Brenda was a 27-year-old single mother with three children (ages 6, 2, and 1). She entered the welfare system when she left an abusive situation and was living in a shelter. Brenda received benefits while attending college. Monica was a 35-year-old single mother with two children (ages 4 and 10). At times, she had worked two jobs to provide for her family. Monica applied for welfare after suffering a series of injuries and life difficulties that made it impossible for her to work; she had received AFDC for about 3 years. Joann was 41 years old and had two children (ages 13 and 20). She was a battered wife and entered the welfare system after leaving her husband. Joann had an extensive employment history and was able to resume working. At the time of the interview, however, she had been laid off and was receiving unemployment compensation.

The selection of these women's voices is deliberate in order to highlight the heterogeneity that is inherent within the population of African American welfare recipients. There is little discussion of this diversity in the popular media. Social scientists, however, have described this heterogeneity using the metaphor of an onion, where the layers represent different subgroups of welfare recipients (Corbett, 1995). The outer layer of the onion represents the working poor who are at risk of requiring welfare, and short-term (less than 2 years) welfare recipients who are thought to enter the program as a result of some discrete and observable adverse circumstance (e.g., divorce or loss of a job). These women have the skills, motivation, and necessary supports to acquire economic self-sufficiency in a short period of time and generally are able to take advantage of the earnings supplements and transitional supports (such as medical coverage and assured childcare) provided by welfare. The middle layer contains women who have limited options for employment and have very low earnings capacity. They tend to remain within the welfare system from 2 to 8 years, but are eventually able to exit from it. The inner core of this metaphorical

---

[1] I would like to give special thanks to Dr. Tracey Spencer, who interviewed three of the women as part of her dissertation research on coping processes in low-income African American single mothers. Dr. Spencer made these transcripts available for reanalysis.

onion represents women who are system dependent, including those with both low earnings capacity and other barriers that impede the way to self-sufficiency (i.e., chemical dependency, clinical depression, and/or abusive personal relations). Also at this layer are those who lack basic skills and who may be isolated from most mainstream institutions. Impoverished neighborhood environments, lack of role models, and inadequate institutional resources contribute to the problems experienced by this core group.

I have chosen to incorporate the voices of women who are more characteristic of those in the upper and middle layers of the metaphorical onion, because their voices are often lost and/or silenced in the public discourse surrounding welfare. As can be seen from the brief descriptions of the four women, there is diversity even within these subgroups. Each of the women entered and exited the welfare system at different phases in their lives and for different reasons, and remained on the welfare rolls for varying lengths of time. Despite this diversity, I believe their experiences illustrate the strength and resistance efforts within this population, and their voices enhance our understanding of the process by which many welfare mothers are able to succeed despite the challenges they face.

In this chapter, I first explore the marginalization of low-income African American mothers through an examination of the more common myths about welfare recipients, and I present data from the research literature that refutes these misconceptions. I next propose an explanation for the development of these negative stereotypes through an analysis of the history of welfare and the changing perceptions of recipients through the years. Finally, I conclude the chapter with a discussion of the ways in which these women have resisted marginalization and overcome the odds against them.

## MYTHS AND REALITY
## ABOUT WELFARE MOTHERS

The popular media is replete with myths about welfare mothers, and the rhetoric associated with welfare reform would have us believe that they are addicted to welfare, destined to remain on aid for more than one generation, unmotivated to escape poverty, and bear children out of wedlock in order to increase the amount of their subsidy. There is also the belief that their dependency on the state leads to (or results from) moral weakness and psychological/pathological dependency

(Spalter-Roth & Hartmann, 1994). These and other myths have led to the recent reforms in the AFDC program. In August 1996, President Clinton signed the welfare reform bill entitled The Personal Responsibility and Work Opportunity Reconciliation Act of 1996. Title I of this Act replaces the federal- and state-funded AFDC program with block grants to states for a new welfare program called Temporary Assistance to Needy Families (Bane, 1997). In essence, this new legislation abolishes any entitlement to benefits and services for poor children and their families, and replaces it with work requirements and a 5-year limit on lifetime eligibility. This new law ends the federally guaranteed cash assistance that was the foundation of the AFDC program and allows each state to shape its own welfare program by determining benefit levels, work mandates, and eligibility requirements. The new legislation seems to ignore the diversity that exists among welfare recipients, and it is questionable whether policy makers will consider this diversity in the development and implementation of state welfare programs. The impact of welfare reform has yet to be realized; however, many have speculated that it will increase the number of children and families living in poverty. The legislation has been passed, and welfare, as we know it, has been abolished; however, it is important to examine the myths that contributed to the public discourse on welfare in the hope that they will no longer have the power to shape policy and to determine the design and implementation of the reformed welfare program.

## Myth 1. Most Women on Welfare Are African American

This myth seems to be the basis for the belief within the larger society that the welfare problem is primarily one that concerns only African Americans. The facts are that the majority of women on welfare are indeed women of color, but most recipients are not African American. Demographic data on the characteristics of welfare recipients indicate that approximately 38% of female recipients are white, 37% are African American, 19% are Latina, 3% are Asian, 1% are Native American, and 2.2% are of unknown ethnicity (U.S. Department of Health and Human Services, 1993). Although their absolute numbers do not place them in the majority on a national level, African Americans are the majority of welfare recipients in a number of states, principally in the South. In these states, the percentages range from 57.4% (Arkansas) to 98.6% (District of Columbia). African American recipients are also overrepresented when compared to their number in the overall population, as indicated by the fact that less than 3% of the white population receives welfare, compared to 17% of African American families (Amott, 1990). These facts, coupled with the racism that continues to exist in this country, have shaped the public perception that African Americans are disproportionately benefiting from welfare—a perception that fueled support for welfare reform.

### Myth 2. Most Women Turn to Welfare When They Have a Baby as a Teenager, and Remain on Assistance for a Long Time

This myth is one of the underlying assumptions supporting the belief that welfare is addictive. Based on actual demographic data, the prototypical welfare recipient is a woman, age 25 years or older, who has at least one child under 6 years old. She is either divorced or separated from the child's father and has, at most, a high school education. The child has one or two siblings, and the family has received welfare for 3 years or less (Green Book, 1994). Monica's entrance into the welfare system was consistent with the above portrait. She had been self-sufficient for 14 years when an unplanned pregnancy led her to welfare. She explained:

> "I've worked for 14 years of my life. My original profession was property management, and I did that for 14 years. When I got pregnant, I did work still. But then I was in a car accident and that made me stop working. So, I haven't worked in about 3 years now. I decided, since I was having a baby and I think it's important for a parent to be home, that I wouldn't work. . . . I have gone through some very, very hard moments to the extent where I just had to get out there and find help. . . . This was before I had the baby. I was pregnant and had to stop working and depleted my savings. And, it was like, what do I do? That's when I went to welfare and applied for public assistance."

Monica and other women like her make the decision to apply for welfare after they have tried other options. For most, it is the solution of "last resort" and one that is not easily chosen because of their awareness of the negative perception of welfare recipients held by society.

About 38% of those entering the welfare system are unmarried women who have just given birth (Berrick, 1991). Although teen mothers have received intense focus in the public discourse on welfare, only 7.5% of all female welfare recipients are under age 20 (U.S. Department of Health and Human Services, 1993). The data also indicate that welfare recipients do not have unusually large families. Overall, there has been a decline in the average family size of welfare recipients, and currently 72.7% of these families have two or fewer children (Green Book, 1994).

The facts also refute the assertion that once on welfare, women tend to remain on the rolls for a long period of time. Data have been collected since the 1960s indicating that more than two-thirds of the individuals on welfare receive assistance for less than 2 years, while over half of these families exit the system in a year or less. For more than 20 years, data have indicated that only a small proportion (12% in 1965 and 17% in 1993) of welfare mothers have periods in their lives where they consistently receive benefits for 8 years or longer (Burgess, 1965; Greenberg, 1993).

The data indicate that many women enter and exit welfare a number of times before they are permanently off it. Of those women who exit through earned income, 40% remain poor; 42% of this number return to welfare within 2 years of leaving it; and 75% of those reentering welfare exit again (Greenberg, 1993; Pavetti, 1993). Carla's experiences were representative of women who have brief periods on welfare interspersed with periods of work:

> "I've been on and off welfare so many times. I first got on it when I was around 5 months pregnant with my daughter, and when she was 3 months I went back to business school. . . . I graduated and then I got a job. . . . I stayed off for 5 years. And then I got pregnant with my son and I was having a real bad relationship with my supervisor at the time, so I wound up having to leave my job and having to go back and apply for welfare because I was 7 months pregnant. There was no way that they were gonna give me unemployment because I couldn't actively look for a job. So, I had to get welfare and I finally got off . . . and ended back on in 1995."

About 15% of the total population of welfare recipients are continuous recipients, and even in these "highly dependent" welfare homes (defined as having 25% or more of the household income coming from welfare payments), on average only one out of four daughters becomes highly dependent herself (U.S. Congress, House Committee on Ways and Means, 1994; Duncan et al., 1988; Furstenburg, 1992). More than three out of five (64%) of the daughters with welfare-dependent backgrounds receive no welfare benefits (Duncan et al., 1988). The stereotype of heavy welfare dependence being passed from mother to child is contradicted by the data. Those families characterized by intergenerational dependency on welfare represent the inner core of our metaphorical onion, and their needs are intense and often remain unmet in the current welfare system. Brenda voiced her opinion about the responsibility she feels the state has in perpetuating this dependency:

"Well, people always blame the welfare recipient and say they should get a job. But nobody ever talks about how the system is addictive, and nobody is doing anything to rehabilitate the welfare system. They threaten them about going to this job search program, but still don't wean them off. They're not rehabilitating them. [The system is] threatening them, and the women are not doing it [job search program] because they want to. They're doing it because their check is in jeopardy, and so that's a real serious complex issue."

Brenda's comments highlight the complexity inherent in the welfare system. The women who are the most needy recipients can, and often do, become psychologically dependent on the receipt of welfare benefits. They have few employable skills and often have been on the welfare rolls for most of their lives as children and adults. Brenda is aware of the pervasive unmet needs of this subgroup of welfare mothers and holds the government accountable. Given the current welfare legislation, the concerns that Brenda expresses are no longer relevant, because all welfare recipients will now be required either to participate in training opportunities or to work in order to receive benefits, and will only be allowed to remain in the welfare program for a limited amount of time. Despite this new legislation, the problems faced by long-term, multigenerational welfare recipients are not easily solved. Welfare reform was in part designed to address the problem of dependency; however, the new legislation appears to underestimate these women's needs for intensive rehabilitation and training. If policy makers are willing to acknowledge the heterogeneous nature of the welfare-recipient population, it may be possible to develop programs that will meet the unique needs of recipients in the different subgroups. If this diversity is ignored, it will most likely lead to programs that provide little assistance to long-term welfare recipients, who will remain at the margins of society and continue to live in pervasive poverty.

## Myth 3. Most Women on Welfare Are Lazy and Do Not Want to Work

The myth surrounding welfare mothers' motivation to work has contributed to changes in welfare regulations requiring mandatory training and/or work as a condition of eligibility; however, over 30 years of research results refute this myth. Since the 1960s, studies have found that many women on welfare have work histories and/or they work while receiving benefits. Burgess and Price (1963) found that 30% worked before receiving welfare, and another 30% combined work and welfare; Podell (n.d.) found that 8 in 10 welfare mothers have work histories; and a Department of Health, Education and Welfare survey conducted in 1969 found that 61% of welfare mothers had been employed prior to receiving benefits (U.S. Congress, House Committee on Ways and Means, 1969).

In a more recent study, Spatler-Roth and Hartmann (1994) found that 4 out of 10 welfare recipients they surveyed reported significant hours of paid employment during the survey period, while one-half of these "work/welfare packagers" received income from family, and 30% received income from child support. They also found that although 57% of mothers were dependent on the state for all of their income, 20% combined work with welfare, and another 23% cycled between work and welfare. The most recent national statistics indicate that 3% of all female welfare recipients work full-time, 4% work part-time, 11% are either laid off or unemployed, and 12% are in job training programs or involved in some form of self-initiated training (U.S. Department of Health and Human Services, 1993). Although the number of welfare recipients in the workforce has declined since the earlier studies, economic conditions have also declined and employment opportunities for all workers have worsened since the 1980s. Nevertheless, the data indicate that a large percentage of female welfare recipients (approximately 30%) are either in the workforce or participating in training programs.

A picture begins to emerge that is different from the one painted by the public discourse. Carla combined working with welfare assistance at many points in her life, and she commented on the dilemma that women face who are heads of household and trying to support themselves and their children:

"A large majority [of women on welfare] have had jobs and been on jobs for a number of years at a time. And I think it's a big decision when a woman says, you know, 'Do I go to work at a dead-end job where I'm not going to advance, stay there for 10 years, and just get a cost of living increase each year? Or, do I go to school and back on welfare?' . . . Having just a job is not gonna make it. I have two mouths I have to feed . . . all along, working, I didn't actually make enough money to live on my own with two kids."

Joann's and Brenda's experiences are representative of those women who have opted to return to welfare while they pursue educational opportunities that will advance them beyond minimum-wage employment:

"When I was married, I was middle class and I had no worries about money. I worked to buy the things I wanted, but I really didn't have to work. . . . Now, as a single mother, I work to provide a living for my children. . . . I went back to school and back on AFDC so that I could get a degree and make the kind of money that I needed to make to maintain the lifestyle that my children were accustomed to when I was married."—JOANN

"School is what's gonna get me out of this hole. Period. And I don't want anything to get in the way of that. I know that my education is gonna get me off of AFDC all together, completely off. . . . I know that whatever job it is that I do, the pay I want to get requires education; it requires a degree of some sort, you know." —BRENDA

Welfare seems to be the last resort for women who no longer have financial support from their spouse or partner and who cannot find work or have lost their jobs. It is also used by women who have decided to pursue higher education in hope of securing better-paid employment in the future. From the comments of Carla, Joann, and Brenda, and the research findings through the years, it seems clear that many women who are welfare recipients do want to work and have worked prior to entering the welfare system, as well as while receiving benefits and during periods when they have been able to exit the system temporarily. The mandatory work requirements that are a component of the new welfare legislation do not seem to be necessary for the many women who characteristically use welfare as a short-term, intermittent source of assistance during difficult times, and it has caused at least some recipients to feel that the government disregards their personal efforts to better their life circumstances.

### Myth 4. Women on Welfare Have Lots of Children and Once on Welfare, They Keep Having Children in Order to Increase Payments

The facts are that, on average, women on welfare have only two children: 42% of recipients have one child, 30% have two children, 16% have three children, and the remaining 12% have four or more children (U.S. Department of Health and Human Services, 1993). As early as the 1970s, researchers found that women on welfare were conscientious about using contraceptives, unlikely to want an additional pregnancy, and unlikely to become pregnant while on welfare (Placek & Hendershot, 1974). This attitude toward childbearing appears to be the same for women in the 1990s, as recent studies have found that women on welfare have lower fertility rates than women in the general population and are less likely to have an additional child than are women not on welfare (Rank, 1992; Abramovitz, 1996).

This myth is also disputed by the fact that women on welfare receive limited funding in most states, and this amount is only marginally increased by the birth of a child. In 1986, only 19 of the 50 states in the United States paid welfare benefits that put a family of three at 50% of the poverty line; the remaining states provided benefits that were even lower (Burtless, 1986). Although the states vary greatly in the amount of the average monthly stipends (ranging from $100.27 in Puerto Rico to $886.10 in Alaska), 34 states provide welfare payments that are at or below the average stipend amount (U.S. Department of Health and Human Services, 1993). In 1993, the average monthly AFDC payment to a family with two children was $380.91, which places the family well below the poverty line. Payments do rise with the birth of each additional child. However, in most states, the average increase in the minimum monthly welfare benefit is only about $70, which scarcely meets the cost of feeding, clothing, housing, and educating that child. Given these facts, there seems to be little financial incentive for women to bear additional children while on welfare.

Carla explained her opinion about this myth:

"You know, it's just a stereotype that women are having babies and they're staying home and not doing anything. And you know, it's beyond me that anyone has a child and they're not doing anything. So that the whole stereotype around that is just totally negative. . . . It wasn't like I decided to have kids and not have a father or a husband around. That was never my decision. You know, you think that he's a wonderful man. So you think everything will work out. And then, things happen."

Carla had not planned to be a single parent, and she did not think about increasing her family's income through having additional children. The facts suggest that her experiences are not unique.

## THE DEVELOPMENT OF THE WELFARE MOTHER STEREOTYPE

In light of these research findings, what could possibly be the motivation for the public attack on African American welfare mothers? I believe that the answer can be found in the history of welfare and the ways in which society has differentiated between the "deserving" and the "undeserving" poor. The institutional response to female poverty began in the late 1800s and early 1900s when suffragettes made women's role in reproduction a political issue, one that entitled them to public support (Mink, 1990). They took the position that the state needed to support women who were without male breadwinners because they were the defenders of moral standards and orderliness within the home. By 1915, 29 states had instituted Mothers' Pensions programs for "deserving" women who were without husbands due to death (Marks, 1991). The ideology reflected in the Mothers' Pensions was that deserving widows (usually white women) who had been deprived of a male breadwinner were entitled to be dependent on the state (Axinn & Hirsch, 1993). This program enabled poor women either to give up work or to cut back on hours worked, so that they could resume their "natural" role of raising responsible citizens for the nation.

In order to receive assistance under this program, a woman was required to maintain a standard of "moral fitness" within her home and could be terminated from the program for "immoral behavior." The assessment of both "moral fitness" and "immoral behavior" was made by the agencies administering the program. In most states, African American and immigrant women were excluded from receiving benefits because they were considered by the program's administrators to have failed the "moral fitness" test due to perceived flaws in their parenting skills, housekeeping, and/or relationships with males (Abramovitz, 1988).

The Mothers' Pension program was expanded in 1935 by legislation that changed the focus of aid from mothers to children. The Aid to Dependent Children (ADC) program provided grants for families headed by mothers who did not have male support, regardless of their status as widows. With the establishment of the Survivor's Insurance program, widows were removed from the ADC program, and only women who were divorced, separated, and/or never married remained. The ADC program was more broad based, which made it somewhat more likely that African American women would be eligible to receive benefits. However, the removal of widows from the program contributed to a public distinction between "good" and "bad" mothers. Widows maintained their positive image, while all other single mothers who were unable either to establish or to maintain two-parent, intact families were considered "bad mothers." By the 1970s, women of color (including a large percentage of African Americans), divorced, and never-married women became the majority of the welfare caseload, and when political conservatives began to attack the program in the 1980s, these women became the focus of the controversy (Gordon, 1990).

The "worthy white widow" halo that had been the prevailing image of the welfare recipient prior to the 1940s had by the 1980s shifted to the "unworthy urban African American woman," and the negative stereotypical image of welfare mothers was born (Axinn & Hirsch, 1993). In place of the moral fitness requirement of the past there was an emphasis on rehabilitation services designed to combat what was thought to be welfare dependency and illegitimacy (Ad Hoc Committee on Public Welfare, 1961). In the eyes of policy makers and the general public, mothers who received welfare were responsible for their own poverty and had to be helped to change their work habits and personal behavior in order to exit the welfare rolls (Axinn & Stern, 1988).

The development of this stereotypical image of African American welfare mothers has taken place within a broader sociopolitical context. During its earlier years, the welfare program (ADC and AFDC) reflected the overt racism that was prevalent in society. In many Southern states, employers and policy makers believed that there was no reason why the employable African American mother should not continue her usual sketchy seasonal labor or indefinite domestic service rather than receive public assistance. Many local welfare departments gave these women less money than they did white women or denied their applications for assistance (Abramovitz, 1996). In later years, welfare policies were influenced by social scientists' portrayal of the urban "underclass." This term was first used in the 1960s to describe a concentrated, isolated population of the urban poor that were thought to be pathological and damaged (Glasgow, 1980). The dependent, African American welfare mother was one of the stereotypical images that emerged from these reports. Policies on poverty resulting from this perspective led conservatives to call for the elimination of welfare and all race-conscious affirmative action programs (Williams, 1992). Welfare mothers had become proxies for the undeserving poor—they stood for themselves and for the absent, unemployed men that society felt should be taking care of them and their children (Williams, 1992).

Thus, the history of welfare and the sociopolitical context surrounding the program have contributed to the stereotypical images and myths that abound in this society about African American welfare mothers. Yet, some women have found ways to resist these negative stereotypes and manage to lead positive and productive lives.

## AGAINST ALL ODDS

There can be little doubt that African American welfare mothers are facing tremendous odds, given the public discourse surrounding welfare, the stereotypes and myths about welfare mothers, and the very real economic obstacles these women face when attempting to support their families. Yet, even within this adverse societal context, welfare mothers have found ways to resist marginalization. Carla's and Joann's comments illustrate the concept of *resistance for equality* (Robinson & Ward, 1991). Carla focused on the rights of welfare recipients:

> "When I was a social worker going into welfare offices with clients . . . it was a depressing experience. Just the whole atmosphere of the place is just so horrendous. And, the workers were rude. . . . It hasn't changed—they still treat you really bad. . . . [Society] wants to take everything from me. They want to take your dignity, your self-esteem, your self-worth, and everything else from you when you're on welfare. . . . We can no longer allow them to do that. . . . I don't know if you actually put up a wall; I think you just try to ignore it. But I can't say it doesn't affect me, because it does. . . . I do have rights and I can fight for myself. . . . We have to stand up and fight for ourselves, regardless of whether

we're getting help from others. . . . They just want us to go away, but we're not going anywhere. That's when we need to say, 'We're not going away, no matter what you do we're not going away.' "

Joann resisted by being assertive and challenging the system. She stated:

"The system itself looks down on you. The welfare system and society, they look upon you as being poor and good for nothing and you don't want anything but the pay check. . . . You don't want to do better and that you are not entitled to the money. . . . I had to fight a lot with them. I wouldn't conform to them."

Comments made by Brenda and Joann illustrate *resistance for survival* (Robinson & Ward, 1991) and draw attention to the personal efforts made by welfare mothers to deal with the negative public perception of welfare recipients and to maintain a sense of positive self-esteem in the face of such stigma. Brenda handled this by remaining "invisible" when she was interacting in a public forum:

"I don't talk about being on welfare because the school I go to is a discussion-type school and in a lot of the classes you discuss issues. People have negative responses about welfare recipients, and I don't talk about it. I don't let on that I'm on welfare."

Reframing is another strategy that the four women interviewed used to resist the effects of negative stereotypes. They found ways to redefine their reliance on welfare that preserved a positive sense of self. Carla stated:

"We know we are somebody regardless of whether we need help or not. You know everybody needs help at some point in their life. And you shouldn't feel like you're the lowest of the low because you need help. . . . I just say to myself, 'No matter what people say, I am somebody and I'm not going to let anyone take that away from me.' "

For Monica, her friends provide the reframe:

"[Friends help] because they say that it's not like you're gonna be on it forever. It's not like this is what you really wanted. These things happen, and you gotta support yourself. You gotta take care of yourself. So they were supportive. They really helped me through a very difficult period because you start losing your self-esteem; you start feeling like this is not what you had planned."

*Resistance for liberation* (Robinson & Ward, 1991) uses collective strategies in order to bring about self-affirmation, self-determination, and community validation. Carla's comments illustrate the need for collective action in dealing with welfare:

"I think more women need to look at welfare reform because it's not just welfare recipients that are affected—it's women in general. . . . I mean, we need to think about the struggle we have had as women, color or no color. I think there is definitely a need for us to come together and fight this fight together because there is almost no way that welfare recipients can do it alone."

Although collective activism may indeed be an effective approach to resistance, many women are not willing (or able) to become involved. Carla often served as an advocate and became frustrated when recipients were unable (or unwilling) to commit themselves to activities (such as group meetings or speaking engagements) that would further the cause for proactive reforms. She said:

"I think it comes down to commitment because what's funny is there are more women who aren't on welfare who are interested in what can be done than women who are on it. And I keep seeing that happen too. They're just sitting back and saying 'OK.' But it's not OK—you can't just keep sitting back and saying OK. . . . The problem is that it's too individualized. They think, 'Oh, as long as I get out of school.' But, what about the next person who's coming in after you that's gonna be struggling. They need all the support. . . . I think it's real important for women, period. I went and did a demonstration down at the State House and a reporter asked me why I was there. I said, first and foremost, because I'm a woman, regardless of whether I'm receiving AFDC or not. And this is a woman's issue."

Women who are experiencing a sense of victimization and have been negatively affected by the poverty and stress in their lives are often unable to engage actively in resistance efforts. Often it is necessary for therapists and other professionals involved in these women's lives to provide this sort of advocacy, while finding ways to further self-empowerment through the provision of information and support.

African American welfare mothers are also aided in their efforts to resist negative stereotypes and marginalization through identifying with role models and developing communities of resistance. Each of the four women interviewed had at least one role model, usually her mother, who had overcome the odds. These women used their role models to maintain a sense of hope that someday, somehow they would achieve self-sufficiency and move beyond the need to rely on welfare. Carla said:

> "I don't know. I just had this vision, you know, if my mother could do it, then I could do it. She was determined. . . . I watched her stay determined and just do what she needed to do to take care of her family. . . . I watched my mother struggle with having us, with going off and on welfare, with trying to get a job."

Brenda and Monica also have similar memories of their mothers:

> "My mother's a really good role model. She was also on AFDC after my father left her. She was on AFDC and she worked a little bit. She decided when I was 15 years old she wanted to go to school and she got a master's degree."—BRENDA

> "I would go back to when I was young and my mom (*pause*) and just thinking about her strength and how strong she was, you know, raising three kids. Just never giving up. . . . My mother was a prime example of someone who could of said, 'I'm gonna let the system take care of me.' But she didn't. She could of, but she didn't. . . . She said, 'When I left your father I had to go on welfare.' I think she said they gave her like $80 or something for like 2 weeks for three kids. It was hard for her."—MONICA

For these three women, their mothers were significant role models and provided examples of how hard work and determination could be successful in enabling a woman to exit the welfare system.

The communities of resistance for these women include family members, friends, and institutional support persons. Previous research has noted that one of the traditional and continuing stress-absorbing systems for African Americans and other minorities has been the wide supportive network of their families (Ball, Warbeit, Vandizer, & Holzer, 1979; McAdoo, 1982; Belle, 1982; Gibbs, 1990). Joann spoke about the support she received from her mother and sister in caring for her children:

> "My mother, when she was alive, was very supportive. She would always take the kids. When my mother died, my sister took up the slack. We just kind of shared in childcare. I would help with her kids when she needed it. . . . I could always depend on her to baby-sit and when the kids became teenagers she helped me with them too."

Brenda and Carla acknowledged the support they received from individuals within institutional systems. This support was perceived as being tremendously helpful and seemed essential in their efforts to maintain a positive sense of self during difficult times. Brenda stated:

> "My advocate was my biggest help. I don't know what I'd do without her. She helped me get this apartment; she helped me get into school . . . she believed in me and gave me this real powerful push."

Carla's support came from college professors:

> "We've had meetings recently around this daycare issue. The faculty at my college said, 'What do you need us to do? What help do you need from us?' And that's really important because our college already stands out from the rest . . . so it's really important that I have faculty support."

It is unclear whether the supports that these two women spoke about are available to most welfare recipients. Both the research findings and my clinical experience with welfare mothers whose life experiences are more characteristic of those at the inner core of the metaphorical onion suggest that such supports are either not readily available to these women or may be experienced as problematic (Wyche & Lobato, 1996). Belle (1984) suggests that for poor women the strain and distress associated with providing support to extended family members may diminish the effectiveness of any help they receive. Indeed, there seem to be some welfare mothers whose stressful lives leave them with very little to give (either emotionally or materially) to others in their extended families. And when resources in kinship networks are similarly depleted, available supports are meager and insufficient to meet mothers' needs.

Jayakody, Chatters, and Taylor (1993) found that even when kin networks are able to provide such supportive functions as childcare and financial assistance, this support is not as prevalent or extensive as had been suggested in previous research. Close to a quarter of never married African American mothers in their large-scale study received financial assistance from family members, but less than a fifth received childcare help. However, emotional support was found to be much more prevalent, with four out of five of these mothers receiving extensive emotional support from kin. In an earlier study, Ball and colleagues (1979) found that low-income African American women were less willing to request help from family and friends, believing that to request help would be admitting defeat and lead to negative evaluations of self. It would appear that receiving support from kinship networks is a complex endeavor, and that it may be neither as prevalent nor as uniformly supportive as has been suggested by some research. The claim that extended family involvement largely mitigates the difficulties faced by African American single mothers seems to overstate the prevalence of aid provided to these women. But, when such support is given, it can help welfare mothers sustain their families and contribute to the maintenance of a positive sense of self in at least some women.

The experiences of Carla, Monica, Brenda, and Joann suggest that African American women who have had periods in their lives on welfare are able to resist the impact of the stereotypical image of welfare mothers. They do so through utilizing such strategies as reframing their experience of dependency in such a way that they are able to preserve a positive sense of themselves, participating in collective activism and advocacy, identifying with role models, and developing communities of resistance through the use of interpersonal and institutional supports.

## IMPLICATIONS FOR MOTHERING

These four women are examples of the many welfare mothers who are struggling against the odds—and succeeding. Their experiences of parenting under economic hardship can further our understanding of the complexities involved in mothering during the 1990s. As these women spoke about mothering and relationships with their children, it became clear that there was closeness and openness in their family communications. Each, to varying degrees, shared her frustrations and survival struggles with her children, both in words and through behaviors that the children observed. Brenda said:

> "One day my oldest son said to me, 'Why don't you just turn us over to DSS [Department of Social Services]. You keep saying you can't do this. . . . I know you can't do this so why don't you just run. You're so good at running.' (*pause*) That was the turning point. I was devastated, and I went through the crying thing, and I sat with myself. . . . Every day I have to be aware of me and my feelings around this issue 'cause I still don't feel like I'm the best parent. But I know I'm the only parent they have."

There was an authenticity within these parental relationships that allowed children to understand and "know" their mothers in ways that are not often experienced within more traditional family structures. These women were "real" to their children, just as their mothers had been real to them. This sort of authenticity between mothers and their children has received some attention in the literature. Weingarten (1997) noted that when a woman is able to create a collaborative, nonhierarchical family structure and to share herself accurately with her partner and children, she, and they, are practicing a form of cultural resistance. The four women interviewed had developed such family structures and were passing on to their own children the valuable lessons about survival that they learned from their own mothers.

The experiences of such welfare mothers are an important source of knowledge for all women, regardless of ethnicity or social class, particularly in light of the fact that most American children will spend at least part of their childhood in a single-parent family (Hamberg, 1992). There will be many women who, at some point in their lives, become single mothers raising children alone. The creative coping responses and richness of family experiences exhibited by this subgroup of mothers can serve as models of how to keep up one's spirits while providing a loving, stable home where authentic relationships exist between family members. These women found ways to resist marginalization and the negative stereotypes that abound in our society. They were resourceful in meeting the challenge of parenting in the midst of poverty, and they learned to be self-reliant (Olson & Ceballo, 1996). We could all learn valuable lessons about survival and mothering from their experiences. This population of women has long been neglected in the research arena; thus, we know far too little about the nature of their families, parenting practices, supportive networks, coping processes, and patterns of exiting welfare. The experiences and voices of African American welfare mothers, along with those of other marginalized groups of mothers, have been ignored and/or excluded from public and scholarly discourse for far too long. If we are to construct a comprehensive conceptualization of mothering in today's society, the voices of African American welfare mothers must be heard.

## REFERENCES

Abramovitz, M. (1988). *Regulating the lives of women: Social welfare policy from colonial times to the present.* Boston: South End Press.

Abramovitz, M. (1996). *Under attack, fighting back: Women and welfare in the United States.* New York: Monthly Review Press.

Ad Hoc Committee on Public Welfare. (1961). *Report to the Secretary of Health, Education and Welfare.* Washington, DC: U.S. Government Printing Office.

Amott, T. L. (1990). Black women and AFDC: Making entitlement out of necessity. In L. Gordon (Ed.), *Women, the state, and welfare.* Madison, WI: University of Wisconsin Press.

Axinn, J. M., & Hirsch, A. E. (1993). Welfare and the "reform" of women. *Families in Society, 74*(9), 563–572.

Axinn, J., & Stern, M. (1988). *Dependency and poverty.* Lexington, MA: Lexington Books.

Ball, R., Warbeit, G., Vandizer, J., & Holzer, C. (1979). Kin ties of low-income Blacks and Whites. *Ethnicity, 6,* 184–196.

Bane, M. J. (1997). Welfare as we might know it. *American Prospect, 30,* 47–53.

Bane, M. J., & Ellwood, D. (1994). *Welfare realities: From rhetoric to reform.* Cambridge, MA: Harvard University Press.

Belle, D. (Ed.). (1982). *Lives in stress: Women and depression.* Beverly Hills, CA: Sage.

Belle, D. (1984). Inequality and mental health: Low income and minority women. In L. Walker (Ed.), *Women and mental health policy.* Beverly Hills, CA: Sage.

Berrick, J. D. (1991). Welfare and child care: The intricacies of competing social values. *Social Work, 36*(4), 345–351.

Burgess, M. E. (1965). Poverty and dependency: Some selected characteristics. *Journal of Social Issues, 21*(1), 79–97.

Burgess, M. E., & Price, D. O. (1963). *An American dependency challenge.* Chicago: APWA Press.

Burtless, G. (1986). Public speaking for the poor: Trends, prospects and economic limits. In S. Danziger & D. Weinberg (Eds.), *Fighting poverty: What works and what doesn't.* Cambridge, MA: Harvard University Press.

Collins, P. H. (1990). *Black feminist thought.* Boston: Unwin Hyman.

Corbett, T. (1995). Why welfare is still so hard to reform. In K. Bogenschneider & T. Corbett (Eds.), *Welfare reform: Can government promote parental self-sufficiency while ensuring the well-being of children?* Madison, WI: Center for Excellence in Family Studies.

Duncan, G. J., Hill, M. S., & Hoffman, S. D. (1988). Dependence within and across generations. *Science, 239,* 467–471.

Fraser, N., & Gordon, L. (1991). *A genealogy of dependency: A keyword of the US welfare state.* Chicago: Center for Urban Affairs and Policy Research, Northwestern University.

Furstenberg, F. (1992). Next generation: The children of teenage mothers grow up. In M. Rosenhelm & M. Teete (Eds.), *Parenthood and coming of age in the 1990s.* New Brunswick, NJ: Rutgers University Press.

Gibbs, J. T. (1990). Developing intervention models for Black families: Linking theory and research. In H. E. Cheatham & J. B. Stewart (Eds.), *Black families: Interdisciplinary perspectives.* New Brunswick, NJ: Transaction Books.

Gilkes, C. T. (1994). If it wasn't for the women. . . . : African American women, community work, and social change. In M. B. Zinn & B. Thorton Dill (Eds.), *Women of color in U.S. society.* Philadelphia: Temple University Press.

Glasgow, D. (1980). *The black underclass: Poverty, unemployment and entrapment of ghetto youth.* San Francisco: Jossey-Bass.

Gordon, L. (Ed.). (1990). *Women, the state, and welfare.* Madison, WI: University of Wisconsin Press.

Greenberg, M. (1993). *Beyond stereotypes: What state AFDC studies on length of stay tell us about welfare as a "way of life."* Washington, DC: Center for Law and Social Policy.

Greene, B. (1994). Diversity and difference: The issue of race in feminist therapy. In M. P. Mirkin (Ed.), *Women in context: Toward a feminist reconstruction of psychotherapy.* New York: Guilford Press.

Hamberg, H. H. (1992). *Today's children: Creating a future for a generation in crisis.* New York: Time Books.

Jayakody, R., Chatters, L. M., & Taylor, R. J. (1993). Family support to single and married African American mothers: The provision of financial, emotional, and child care assistance. *Journal of Marriage and the Family, 55,* 261–276.

Marks, C. (1991). The urban underclass. *Annual Review of Sociology, 17,* 445–466.

McAdoo, H. P. (1982). Stress absorbing systems in black families. *Family Relations, 31*(4), 479–488.

Mink, G. (1990). The lady and the tramp: Gender, race, and the origins of the American welfare state. In L. Gordon (Ed.), *Women, the state, and welfare.* Madison, WI: University of Wisconsin Press.

Olson, S. L., & Ceballo, R. E. (1996). Emotional well-being and parenting behavior among low-income single mothers: Social support and ethnicity as contexts of adjustment. In K. F. Wyche & F. J. Crosby (Eds.), *Women's ethnicities: Journeys through psychology.* Boulder, CO: Westview Press.

Pavetti, L. A. (1993). *The dynamics of welfare and work: Exploring the process by which women work their way off welfare.* Unpublished dissertation, Harvard University, Cambridge, MA.

Placek, P. J., & Hendershot, G. E. (1974). Public welfare and family planning: An empirical study of the "brood sow" myth. *Social Problems, 21,* 660–673.

Podell, L. (n.d.). *Families on welfare in New York City.* New York: Center for the Study of Urban Problems, City University of New York.

Rank, M. R. (1992). The blending of quantitative and qualitative methods in understanding childbearing among welfare recipients. In J. F. Gilgun, K. Daly, & G. Handel (Eds.), *Qualitative methods in family research.* Newbury Park, CA: Sage.

Robinson, T., & Ward, J. V. (1991). A belief in self far greater than anyone's disbelief: Cultivating resistance among African American female adolescents. In C. Gilligan, A. G. Rogers, & D. L. Tolman (Eds.), *Women, girls, and psychotherapy: Reframing resistance.* New York: Harrington Park Press.

Spalter-Roth, R., & Hartmann, H. I. (1994). Dependence on men, the market, or the state: The rhetoric and reality of welfare reform. *Journal of Applied Social Sciences, 18*(1), 55–70.

Sparks, E. (1996). Overcoming stereotypes of mothers in the African American context. In K. F. Wyche & F. J. Crosby (Eds.), *Women's ethnicities: Journeys through psychology.* Boulder, CO: Westview Press.

U.S. Congress, House, Committee on Ways and Means. (1969, October 17). *Report of findings of special review of Aid to Families with Dependent Children in New York City.* Washington, DC: U.S. Government Printing Office.

U.S. Congress, House Committee on Ways and Means. (1994). *Overview of entitlement programs, 1994 green book.* Washington, DC: U.S. Government Printing Office.

U.S. Department of Health and Human Services. (1993). *Characteristics and financial circumstances of AFDC recipients.* Washington, DC: U.S. Government Printing Office.

Weingarten, K. (1997). *The mother's voice: Strengthening intimacy in families.* New York: Guilford Press. (Originally published 1994 by Harcourt Brace)

Williams, B. (1992). Poverty among African Americans in the urban United States. *Human Organization, 51*(2), 164–174.

Wyche, K. F., & Lobato, D. (1996). Minority mothers: Stress and coping when your child is in special education. In K. F. Wyche & F. J. Crosby (Eds.), *Women's ethnicities: Journeys through psychology.* Boulder, CO: Westview Press.

# 11

## Teen Mothers
### Countering the Myths of Dysfunction and Developmental Disruption

PATRICIA FLANAGAN

As a pediatrician, I have worked with very young teen mothers for 10 years. I provide primary health care for these young parents and their infants through the Teens with Tots Program, which is located in a tertiary medical center. The program is multidisciplinary with a strong social work focus and liaison to area schools and vocational programs. There is also an emphasis on providing contraception and information about sexual decision making in order to prevent future unwanted pregnancies.

During these same 10 years, I have also begun my own adventures in parenting. My children are now 7, 8, and 9 years old. Thus, much of my own development as a parent has been woven through my experiences working with teen mothers. I recognize commonalities in our experiences as well as stark contrasts. I am intrigued by adolescence, an exciting, challenging, and dynamic developmental stage. Working with adolescents who are also new parents has proven to be intellectually and emotionally rewarding, albeit sometimes frustrating.

I began working in the Teens with Tots Program as a fellow in an academic medical center, having been trained to think about adolescent behavior and misbehavior in a holistic way. One prevailing notion at the time (from the 1970s on) was that dysfunctional behaviors clustered together. Certainly early pregnancy and parenthood were considered dysfunctional behaviors, on a par with other types of acting-out behaviors such as substance abuse, alcohol abuse, interpersonal violence, truancy, and running away. This view is still very prevalent in the conceptualization of youth as "high risk" (Jessor, 1991; Jessor & Jessor, 1977; Zabin, 1984).

The young women with whom I worked were all under 16 when they delivered their first baby. All of them were inner city, poor youths. They were also a culturally and ethnically heterogeneous group. As I continued to work with them, I was struck by their individuality, their unique stories, motivations, and decision-making processes, and by the clumsy, fragile self-image of some and the incredible strength of others. Through listening to, watching, and interacting with these young women, I began to understand early pregnancy not as a dysfunctional behavior or part of a constellation of dysfunctional behaviors but as, sometimes, an alternative developmental pathway; sometimes a rational option, sometimes a shifting of life course, but always a complex, individually experienced event. Each young woman embarks on early motherhood under her own unique set of circumstances, motivations, assumptions about her world and her future, and her own personal experiences with mothers and motherhood. Focus on the "problem" of teen childbearing as unidimensionally negative obscures and denies the complexity of how each individual ended up pregnant and chose to give birth and raise her children.

In this chapter, I argue that much of what mediates the impact of these young women's motherhood experiences are developmental processes. In other words, given that adolescence is a stage of development where individual differences in rate, progression, and growth in the social, emotional, and cognitive realms are immense, these processes have tremendous impact on teenage mothers and their babies. My position is that by paying attention to and increasing our understanding of the ways these processes affect decision making, meaning making, and reactions to the outside world, we can create more individually oriented and, I hope, more effective prevention and intervention programs for these young women and their families. Only then will we be in the position of ameliorating the negative consequences for the mother, the child and society of adolescents having children.

## WHAT IS THE "PROBLEM" OF TEENAGE MOTHERHOOD?

Is teenage pregnancy and motherhood automatically and uniformly dysfunctional? Let us begin by putting current facts and statistics into perspective. Contrary to what the public debate seems to suggest, birth rates to teen mothers were highest in this country in the late 1950s and early 1960s. In each of those decades, approximately 90 in every 1,000 girls in the 15- to 19-year age range became pregnant and gave birth to a child (National Center for Health Statistics, 1990). These numbers consistently declined through the 1960s and 1970s. Rates reached a plateau in the 1980s; currently, we have a slight increase in numbers. However, we are still far below the levels of the early 1960s. In 1993, there were 58 births per 1,000 girls in the 15- to 19-year age range (Annie E. Casey Foundation, 1996).

Another source of confusion is the fact that the terms "school-age mother" and "teenage mother" are often used interchangeably. Yet current statistics show that most teenage mothers are not school-age mothers. They are mostly 18-, 19-, and 20-year-old young women. For example, in 1993, there were 497,000 babies born to teenagers in this country. Two-thirds of them were born to women who were 18–20 years old (Annie E. Casey Foundation, 1996). The impact of early childbearing for these young women is far less detrimental than for the smaller group of truly school-age mothers. Moreover, across many societies and historical periods, this age range seems to be normative for childbearing.

Another argument is that many of these pregnancies are due to the fact that there is an increasing number of teenagers having sex before getting married. But, actually, sex before marriage is not a particularly new social trend in this country. Studies of church records from two 18th-century New England towns reveal close to 40% of first births occurring within 8 months of marriage, suggesting they were conceived prior to the wedding (D'Emilio & Freedman, 1988). It is childbirth outside of marriage that is the more recent trend.

Thus the "problem" is not necessarily having a child at an early age or getting pregnant before marriage, but doing it (getting pregnant and raising a child) out of wedlock. However, this trend is not only observed among teenage mothers. Rates of birth to unmarried mothers have indeed climbed dramatically over the past 20 years. This rise, though, has been most dramatic among those in the 20- to 24-year and 24- to 29-year age ranges, not among those in their teenage years (National Center for Health Statistics, 1990). However, it is true that when teenagers give birth, there is a higher probability that they will be unmarried.

In addition, social science research also suggests that raising a child without the financial advantage of a two-parent arrangement puts single mothers at risk for living in poverty. That risk is heightened if the single mother has not finished school and acquired the vocational skills necessary to support a family. The probability of getting a high school diploma is far lower if she has a child before she finishes high school (Maynard, 1996). It is even more of a problem for very young teen mothers who are perhaps in the seventh or eighth grade when they deliver their first child. Therefore, the "problem" of teenage pregnancy derives primarily from the economic and family circumstances of the mother.

Given the picture so far, it might seem logical to conclude that teenage motherhood leads to poverty, but this conclusion would be naive and simplistic. Teen pregnancy and childbearing are not random events. Children who are already poor are more likely to begin their childbearing at a younger age than children who are not poor. This is an even greater likelihood for children living in socioeconomically segregated communities such as African Americans and Latinos (Henshaw & Van Vort, 1989).

When young mothers have difficulty finishing school, is the difficulty caused by motherhood? Perhaps not. Girls who are struggling in school as early as fourth and fifth grade are at a greater risk for early childbearing than their counterparts who are successful in the educational system (Dryfoos, 1990; Holden, Nelson, Velasquez, & Ritchie, 1993; Rauch-Elnekave, 1994). Thus, even before they have children, those girls who become adolescent mothers are at greater risk than the general population not to finish school and to be poor as adults. It is not the act of childbearing that makes them poor. Does it contribute to keeping them poor? Probably it does. Very young teen mothers may be at considerable risk for poor life outcomes (Maynard, 1996), but it may be a false assumption that the early pregnancy is the cause of this. Rather, the early pregnancies are a response to these girls' perceptions of, and the reality of, their life options (Dodson, 1996).

## BEYOND VICTIMS AND VILLAINS: THE PREVALENT MYTHS OF MOTIVATION

The prevalent misconceptions about the "problem" of teenage mothers are also seen in the explanations of why "unmarried, poor teenagers keep on having children" (García Coll & Vazquez García, 1996). My experience is that there are a multitude of causes for early childbearing, and yet there remains a tendency in the public discourse to simplify the issue.

One of these oversimplifications is the tendency to view the events solely in terms of personal choice and irresponsibility. Teen mothers pushing their scarlet letters in fancy strollers are seen as having made a mistake. They are unmarried. They are poor. They are underage. They are seen as "bad." They have chosen the wrong road out of so many options and resources being put in front of them by the rest of us.

Not surprisingly, many of these messages are internalized, sometimes contributing to a further narrowing of life options for these young women. A sense of failure develops, a belief that one has "doomed" oneself because of early parenthood. It is not uncommon to hear young mothers speak of their "mistakes" while they are also clearly indicating that their pregnancies and subsequent childbearing were wanted and even, at times, planned. The following quotations suggest these young women's struggles in resisting these messages from society:

> "I'm not gonna be what people think. Well, you know, just have babies one after the other, just another black girl sitting on welfare. I want to git me an education and a job."—TOYA, 17 years

> "Um . . . just if teenage moms are gonna, if they wanna have sex, have unprotected sex, and they're gonna have kids, they better make sure the father and them are in a good relationship, that they both want the child and that they have enough money to raise a child, because just about anybody, the majority of teenagers who have kids today, they just go on welfare. You know, that's taking it from people who really need it. They think they'll just have the baby and get on welfare. You know, that's the one thing I say, I don't like welfare and I'm trying to get off it, because I want to be able to give my children what comes out of my pocket, not what comes out of someone else's."—DAWN, 16 years

> "But it wasn't just that, you know, my mother said I should keep it too, because it was my fault and his that I got pregnant, there's no way to kill a baby. And then I started thinking, 'When the baby is born it's not his fault he's gotta go see other parents; he should see his real mother.' And then I started getting ready, and my mother helped me out. She said, 'Are you gonna keep it?' and I said, 'Yeah.' 'Cause it ain't the baby's fault, it's my fault."
> —DEBBIE, 15 years

As evident in these quotes, the cultural conditioning reflected in the language of mistakes exists alongside their own more positive and optimistic subjective experience.

Another source of misrepresentation of these young women's motivations is expressed along racial lines. Solinger (1992) describes a dichotomy in American mythology surrounding sexuality and single childbearing for black and white girls in the 1950s and 1960s. As the myth went, white unmarried girls got pregnant because of deep psychological dysfunction. Black girls, on the other hand, supposedly got pregnant because of a biologically inherent insatiable sex drive. There was a notion that it was somehow more "natural" for young black girls to have babies early, while white girls who did must be mentally disturbed. Such racial stereotyping serves as one more way in which the dominant culture isolates teen mothers, one more reason they are "other" . . . they are not like us. Teen mothers of either race are seen here as either frightening, out-of-control, and immoral, or pitiably flawed in some basic way.

Painting teen mothers always as villains or as victims negates their individual realities and marginalizes their subjective experience. Some young mothers certainly are victims of older males, easy prey to experienced predators (Males & Chew, 1996; Taylor, 1997); or victims of early sexual abuse who now want to gain attention and/or affection through sex (Rainey, Stevens-Simon, & Kaplan, 1995; Stevens-Simon & Reichert, 1994). Many are victims of poverty and of a paucity of life options (Dodson, 1996).

Yet, each has her own set of life circumstances and conscious and subconscious motivations for early parenthood. Some are responsible young women striving to create a life and a family. Others might have the wish and not the means to accomplish such goals. In recognizing their individuality and circumstances, we can reinforce their resistance to being seen as myths that do not represent their real-life experiences. Perhaps more importantly we can help them find ways to build on their individual strengths to optimize their own developmental outcomes and the outcomes of their children.

## SOCIAL INCENTIVES
## FOR TEEN MOTHERHOOD

There is a complex interplay between the motivations for or against pregnancy and for or against childbearing. This interplay is linked to the position of childbearing in the life course. The full range of these motivations warrant our consideration. A few young women do become pregnant because of ignorance. A few do so because of a developmental inability to relate cause and effect, or an inability to think and plan in an abstract way. A few also get pregnant because birth control or contraception is not available or they did not trust it or using it would make public that they were sexually active. However, in my experience, many more girls get pregnant because there are positive incentives for it and very little motivation against it.

The status of motherhood itself is an important motivation in favor of pregnancy. A mother is someone with a job, a role, and a clear, solid identity. A mother has great responsibility and authority. Mothering gives a clear purpose to life. Childbearing also raises a girl's status quickly from child to adult. This route to adulthood is attainable and available. It is a way to become like one's own mother, sisters, and cousins.

A baby can also be an incentive in itself. It is one's own to have, to love, and to teach. Bearing children also is a way of showing your partner that you are committed to him. It is something to give a boyfriend. Finally, in a fatalistic community, which many of our poor communities are, it assures continuity. It is knowing you will leave something behind when you're not sure you're going to be there.

Teenage childbearing can be a rational choice within the context of poverty and limited (real or perceived) opportunities (Dodson, 1996). Even so, the reader might ask, is it really good for the child, or for the mother? In the real world of many teen mothers, the answer to this question is not a foregone conclusion. Many teens have become mothers because they reasonably anticipate the answer to be: "Yes, it will be good for both mother and child."

In my own work as a pediatrician, I have been struck by the wide range of motivations and competencies that I have encountered among these young mothers. I have found that teenage mothers, even young ones, can be good mothers with healthy children if they have the resources they need. However, they often do need special resources.

## JUGGLING MOTHERHOOD AND ADOLESCENCE: WHAT IS NEEDED TO MAKE IT WORK?

In order to provide effective resources for teenage mothers and their children, we have to ask ourselves what particular resources do teenage mothers need in order to have a good outcome? Are there specific characteristics of adolescents that put them or their children at risk that need to be addressed in prevention and intervention programs? The answer to these questions will vary depending on each individual teen, her level of maturity, her social context, and the social supports available to her.

I would like to propose that the unique developmental qualities of very young mothers are critical influences on the ways in which they experience their new role and their infant. Several salient characteristics of adolescence can permeate their parenting experience. Chronological age in adolescence is only a rough and imprecise indication of cognitive, sexual, and psychosocial maturity. Therefore, the adolescent's own unique developmental status is the real determining factor.

Adolescents can be egocentric. Adolescence is a time for exploration of possibilities, and for establishing and reestablishing relationships with family and peers. It is a dynamic, romanticizing period in which there can be an experimental trying on of new selves, old selves, and other selves. It is a time for finding connections and reconnections to mother and to grandmother, connections to other adult women, and connections to the feminine ideal. It is about loss of confidence and gains in confidence. It is a time of idealism and moralism, righteousness and vulnerability.

Adolescents show a wide range of cognitive abilities, as they become concrete reality-based thinkers, daydreamers, planners, or doers. Adolescent parents are any of these, and sometimes they are all of these. However, it is probably safe to say that developmental issues are more immediate and influential among the younger teenage mothers, who might be closer to middle childhood. Developmental issues permeate the motivation for pregnancy and decision making during pregnancy and parenting. The developmental complexities of adolescence and the challenges of motherhood converge in these very young mothers. At the same time, there is wide variability in the cognitive skills that young people use to navigate this time in the life cycle. Motherhood requires patience, anticipation of the future, and consistency. The skills needed can tax the abilities of adolescents, and their own development can constrain their parenting. But is this the case for all adolescents?

## LISTENING TO TEEN MOTHERS

About 3 years ago, some of the staff of the Teens with Tots Clinic (myself, the program's social worker, or the social work intern) began to ask girls what they thought about mothers and motherhood. Our purpose was to begin to explore the interface of adolescent development and the perception of the maternal role from the mother's point of view. The young women we spoke with were all mothers, they ranged in age from 13 to 18 years, and they all had at least one child, and many had more than one.

During the 3 years, we have, with their permission, conducted over 100 interviews, many of which were audio- or videotaped. Interviews were done in small groups and individually. Subsequently, a semistructured interview with five questions was developed (Flanagan, McGrath, Meyer, & García Coll, 1995). We asked what qualities are characteristic of good mothers and, specifically, what motherhood meant in their own lives.

Content analyses by one of us blind to the chronological age of the mother resulted in classifying the mothers into three groups. This classification was based on the cognitive abilities displayed by the mother in the language she used in describing herself. The three groups—young, middle, and late adolescence—correspond to current conceptualizations of adolescent development (Erikson, 1968), and adolescents can be in any one of the three stages regardless of their chronological age. However, the concept of stages is used here heuristically, not as bounded, stable characteristics of a particular individual because individuals may vacillate between stages.

### Young Adolescence

As we noted earlier, across the interviews we found a full range of cognitive and psychosocial development. Some girls were at a very early stage of development. They were extremely concrete in their perceptions of themselves and their children; they had little future orientation and minimal insight. For these young mothers, motherhood was a "nuts-and-bolts," task-oriented job. It was characteristically described in terms of things you do.

For instance, Debbie was a young mother whose infant was born at home, about 2 months early. She met with us frequently during the 8 weeks that her infant daughter was in the neonatal intensive care unit. She was 15 years old, poor, and white, and she giggled nervously. She planned on moving in with her boyfriend and his mother when the baby was discharged.

In response to the question "Tell me about mothers. What are some characteristics of a good mother?," Debbie answered:

"Well, ya gotta love babies and take care of them . . . like they need proper care. Making sure they have heat, light, a house, food . . . and clothing. She's gonna need it."

When asked if she had ever thought of herself as a mother, Debbie responded:

"I guess . . . I know I'm gonna be a good mother. She's gonna be one spoiled little kid. She's gonna give me a hard time when she grows up. I already see that. Everyone is always getting her things. . . . You gotta make sure she gets all her needles, so she get no diseases. You gotta remember all this. She'll get physicals when she needs them. All this stuff, you gotta remember all this stuff now."

Toya was a beautiful, tall, proud African American girl whose baby was born on her 17th birthday. When asked what makes a good mother, she was thoughtful and measured in her responses as exemplified below:

"It's a hard question, but I think I can answer it. Well, a good mother should be able to take care of herself and her kids and stay away from stuff she don't need, drugs and all that stuff, and other unwanted kids. Take care of them well, make sure your kid is eating and everything, and has good health, getting their shots when they're supposed to, you know. If they're sick, call the doctor and stuff like that."

We define developmental status according to the language used to describe the self during the interview process. It is our argument, then, that for these teen mothers, the same language (a reflection of their cognitive status) will be used in their interpretation of their world, including their motherhood. As such, for both Debbie and Toya being a "good" mother involves practicalities like providing food, clothing, shelter, and basic health care. They are both concrete and egocentric, which puts them at a similar developmental level. Their thinking reflects their individual stage, which is that found in a normal young adolescent. They will not be magically transformed into adults by 9 months of pregnancy.

Yet when adolescent parents act like adolescents, they often defy conventional societal standards of how mothers should act and think. They are labeled a "problem," rather than a person who needs support in her own growth. Developmentally young mothers, like Debbie and Toya, have unique needs, which must be met if outcomes detrimental to both mother and child are to be avoided.

The recognition of the developmental stage not only helps define the needs of adolescent parents, but also the kinds of resources that we as clinicians can provide. Early adolescent parents require help with tasks such as making an environment physically safe for a toddler and budgeting a month's income so there is money for diapers by the end of the month. But these needs do not automatically make them bad parents. Like all parents, developmentally young teenage parents need adequate support in terms of information and guidance. They need physical, emotional, educational, and financial help. Moreover, these needs must be addressed in ways that are sensitive to this developmental status. Language should be simple, direct, and concrete. Abstract concepts should be made as concrete as possible.

### Middle Adolescence

As personal development progresses, descriptions of motherhood and mothering take on a more three-dimensional quality: An affective component begins to appear—there is a relationship with the baby, yet there is a strong egocentric flavor to these descriptions as well. Descriptions of self reflect the daydreaming, unrealistic, and romanticizing qualities of middle adolescence.

For example, Wilma was a 15-year-old Latina. She was finishing her sophomore year in high school and planning to marry her son's father when she graduated. We asked her what are some characteristics of a good mother. Wilma replied:

> "Being a good mother is, like, when you take good care of your baby, and you're always there for him no matter what, and you teach him, teach him what is right and wrong and you're not always partying, going out and stuff, and your baby comes first."

We then asked her what had been the best part about being a mother. Wilma responded:

> "I have someone to talk to, although he doesn't understand yet, after class I just hug him and, you know, play with him and, you know, he makes me happy. "

Wilma's thinking reflects the developmental stage of middle adolescence. The baby's needs become more abstract in nature (e.g., learning), prioritizing is recognized as the conflicting demands are accepted and understood, and the relationship with the child becomes more salient, yet it is defined in terms of the mother's own needs. Middle adolescents often need to be refocused, given insight into a child's individuality, abilities, and needs. Although hopes, dreams and fantasies are important, these mothers sometimes need to be grounded, brought back to reality, and walked through logical steps to plan and complete tasks.

### Late Adolescence

Girls with a more typical late-adolescent sense of self have an ability to think abstractly, discuss feelings, and have insight into self and situations. These girls are able to offer a much richer and fuller description of motherhood. We found an awareness of responsibility and a clearer sense of being engaged in a dynamic relationship with one's child or children.

Tammy was a bubbly, engaging 15-year-old African American woman. She had a 5-month-old infant and lived with her baby's father and her younger sister whom she had raised. In answer to our question about what makes a good mother, she said:

"You know, to love your child, and to be patient. It helps to be patient. And being a teenage mother, I think the most important thing is to love your child. Make sure you got your priorities straight. You're not supposed to give up your life. But you have to remember that everything you do affects your child. That's the hard part."

Dawn, a 16-year-old, was a shy, quiet white girl who had a 9-month-old child and had recently found out she was pregnant again. She had been living on the streets for the past 2 years after running away from an abusive stepfather. Her definition of a good mother was as follows:

"Somebody who is there for their kids at all times. Really, that's it. Because you know what your children need, you know and understand them. Because anyone can have a baby. I just think the main thing about being a mother is being there for them. You know,

it's not just paying the bills or anything. You gotta make sure
you're there for them when they need you. That's basically it."

Young mothers who are developmentally in late adolescence present a more abstract, complex, and realistic description of motherhood.
There are both rewarding and demanding aspects to being a mother.
Their relationships with their children and responding to the varying
needs as they grow up become central in these mothers' conceptualization of motherhood. They can sometimes benefit from more abstract
discussions of roles and life course, and from reflection on their own
lives and different roles as mothers, daughters, friends, and workers.
They may need help in obtaining the education and training required
to reach the goals they have set for themselves, and support in clarifying
their vision for themselves and their children.

## TEEN MOTHERHOOD AS A GIFT

The previous stories have focused on the special needs created for
adolescents by motherhood. But motherhood can also bring special
benefits. For some young mothers, the event of an early birth serves as
a positive developmental force, a focus for positive growth. It is not
unusual to hear of beneficial life trajectory changes wrought by early
motherhood. When we asked mothers to talk a little about ways in
which life has changed since becoming a mother, several answered as
follows:

> "It's changed a lot. First of all, you kinda mature faster, you gotta
> get used to being a mom, get used to being a wife at the same
> time. You can't go out with your friends, you know. Everything
> revolves around your kid. Not so much your house or even your
> husband, but your kid . Everything revolves around the baby."
> —SHARON, 15 years

> "I would like to finish school first of all, 'cause I think that without
> finishing school, you can't go nowhere. Then it will be hard for
> myself and the baby too. I want to be able to give her a nice
> example of myself, and I'll raise her in a good way. Maybe she'll
> take after me. I'd like to finish school for her sake. But I'm gonna
> try to do my best."—ALMA, 16 years

"It changed me because, you know, she got me into school, more interested in school now than I was before. She makes me feel I have a responsibility to somebody, not just myself or my mother anymore, but somebody that belongs to me, you know."—TOYA, 17 years

"I have changed, I know I have. I'm, like, settled down now. She made me settle and focus on my business, you know. I can't be hangin' with those old friends no more, you know. I got different friends now anyway, mostly my cousins and them."—BARBARA, 16 years

Perhaps early motherhood, in poor settings, acts as a kind of social safety valve, a possibility when nothing else is possible. It provides a route that is far safer than the roads to adulthood that many young men and other young women in the same communities are taking, that is, routes of crime, incarceration, and violent interpersonal confrontations.

For some girls then, early pregnancy and parenting connects them with resources within their families, communities, and among their peers. It is a comfortable, familiar role for young women to take. They fit in. They gain support from families and peers for whom early parenting is normative. In many instances the emotional cost of not partaking in early childbearing is high (Dash, 1989; Musick, 1993), leading to other, more destructive pathways into adulthood.

We asked Tammy, 15, several questions about the impact of motherhood on her friendships. For example, had her friendships changed at all since her daughter was born?

"All my close friends have kids. Because my best friend, she was my best friend before, we wasn't friends over the summer 'cause we had a fight or something, and then we came back to school and we were both pregnant. So that just happened. And now it seems like, well mostly every friend that I meet who I get close to already has children or else gets pregnant."

When asked if she still spends time with her friends, she replied:

"Well, we usually go over somebody's house and just sit around and let our kids play together. Once in a while I go out without her. But then I feel guilty when I leave her home or something and

I'm having fun. I miss her so much and I don't wanna go out, I'd rather take her with me."

We asked Dawn, 16, about her relationships with girl friends, and if she still sees them. She answered:

"Oh yeah! and we can understand what each other is going through. 'Cause we all have kids. It's a lot easier when you have friends that have kids. When you don't have kids you don't understand. You know, they say they understand, but they really don't know what you're going through. "

For Wilma, 15, her mother is her main support:

"When I found out I was pregnant, it wasn't so bad, like part of me really wanted to have a baby, but then again I'd think about we're still young, we're still young, I have my whole life ahead of me. But when I found out, I was, like, I was happy and I was, like, we'll have to take it from here. So I told my mom about it. She was the only one giving me my resource. She wasn't upset 'cause me and my mom are best friends, and we really help each other out. So, she just, my mom is real supportive, she just helps me out a lot. And, um, it hasn't been so bad ever since."

For some young women, motherhood is a sign of wholeness and completion. Fertility defines femininity:

"I never used protection. Never. I mean I couldn't, you know. I was scared to go ask the nurse or something. But I thought I probably couldn't get pregnant anyway, you know, having sex all that time and not getting pregnant. Maybe I was really a man, you know, somehow way inside."—MARY, 18 years

## CONCLUSION

Each of the young women I have met and worked with through the Teens with Tots Program has her own unique strengths, her own barriers to overcome, and her own personal history to build on. We as a society and as service providers have to recognize that adolescent mothers are adolescents *and* mothers. These are two simple facts often lost among considerations of problem statistics or societal ills.

We also have to recognize that most portrayals in the media and the research and clinical literature on teenage mothers concentrate on the negative consequences for the children and society at large. Although these portrayals do capture the experience of some teenage mothers and their children, they fail to grasp the complexity of these families' life choices and alternatives. They marginalize their experiences and lead to interventions that are either punitive or insensitive to their more critical needs.

Adolescent parents need the same things that most parents need and the things that most adolescents need for healthy development: the support of extended families and the scaffolding of extended and collective parenting. Adolescent parents need to continue their travels through adolescence while they parent. They need strong communities that nurture young people whether or not they are parenting, communities that provide role models not only for healthy parenting and but also for realistic, attainable alternatives to early parenting.

Honoring these young women's definitions of motherhood, and recognizing them as reflections of their own developmental maturity, will lead to a different understanding of their needs and the resources necessary to meet them. Personal growth and development is a complex process that involves not only individuals, but the relationships and the contextual demands and supports given to these individuals. Until we recognize their unique developmental needs as adolescents and as mothers, adolescent motherhood will be the "problem" that never goes away.

## REFERENCES

Annie. E. Casey Foundation. (1996). *Kids count data book.* Baltimore, MD: Author.

Dash, L. (1989). *When children want children: The urban crisis of teenage childbearing.* New York: Morrow.

D'Emilio, J. & Freedman, E. (1988). *Intimate matters: A history of sexuality in America.* New York: Harper & Row.

Dodson, L. (1996). *"We could be your daughters": Girls, sexuality and pregnancy in low-income America.* Cambridge, MA: Radcliffe Public Policy Institute.

Dryfoos, J. (1990). *Adolescents at risk.* New York: Oxford University Press.

Erikson, E. (1968). *Identity, youth, and crisis.* New York: Norton.

Flanagan, P., McGrath, M., Meyer, E., & García Coll, C. (1995). Adolescent development and the concept of motherhood. *Pediatrics, 96,* 273–277.

García Coll, C., & Vazquez García, H. (1996). Definitions of competence during adolescence: Lessons from Puerto Rican adolescent mothers. In D. Cichetti & S. L. Toth (Eds.), *Rochester Symposium on Developmental Psychopathology: Vol. 7. Adolescence: Opportunities and challenges.* Rochester, NY: University of Rochester Press.

Henshaw, S., & Van Vort, J. (1989). Teenage abortions, birth, and pregnancy statistics. *Family Planning Perspectives, 21,* 85–88.

Holden, G. W., Nelson, P. B., Velasquez, J., & Ritchie, K. L. (1993). Cognitive, psychological, and reported sexual behavior differences among pregnant and nonpregnant adolescents. *Adolescence, 28*(111), 557–572.

Jessor, R. (1991). Risk behavior in adolescence: A psychosocial framework for understanding and action. *Journal of Adolescent Health, 12,* 579–605.

Jessor, R., & Jessor, S. L. (1977). *Problem behaviors and psychosocial development.* New York: Academic Press.

Males, M., & Chew, K. S. (1996). The ages of fathers in California adolescent births, 1993. *American Journal of Public Health, 86*(4), 565–568.

Maynard, R. (Ed.). (1996). *Kids having kids: A Robin Hood Foundation special report on the cost of adolescent childbearing.* New York: Robin Hood Foundation.

Musick, J. (1993). *Young, poor and pregnant: The psychology of teenage motherhood.* New Haven, CT: Yale University Press.

National Center for Health Statistics. (1990). *Advance report on final natality statistics* (Vol. 39, No. 4, Suppl.). Hyattsville, MD: U.S. Department of Health and Human Services.

Rainey, D. Y., Stevens-Simon, C., & Kaplan, D. W. (1995). Are adolescents who report prior sexual abuse at high risk for pregnancy? *Child Abuse and Neglect, 19*(10), 1283–1288.

Rauch-Elnekave, H. (1994). Teenage motherhood: Its relationship to undetectable learning problems. *Adolescence, 29*(113), 92–103.

Solinger, R. (1992).*Wake up little Susie: Single pregnancy and race before Roe v. Wade.* New York: Routledge.

Stevens-Simon, C., & Reichert, S. (1994). Sexual abuse and adolescent pregnancy. *Archives of Pediatric and Adolescent Medicine, 148,* 23–27.

Taylor, D., Chavez, G., Chambra, A., & Boggess, J. (1997). Risk factors for adult paternity in births to adolescents. *Obstetrics and Gynecology, 89*(2), 199–205.

Zabin, L. S. (1984). The association between smoking and sexual behavior among teens. *American Journal of Public Health, 74,* 261–323.

# 12

🐝

# Incarcerated Mothers
## Crimes and Punishments

CYNTHIA GARCÍA COLL
JANET L. SURREY
PHYLLIS BUCCIO-NOTARO
BARBARA MOLLA

For imprisoned mothers, one of the greatest
punishments incarceration carries with it is the
separation from their children. Separation is
antithetical to the development of parental
responsibility. As one mother puts it, "I can do
time alone OK. But it's not knowing what's
happening to my son that hurts most."
—PHYLLIS JO BAUNACH, *Mothers in Prison*
(1988, p. 121)

THE majority of women in prison are mothers. In many profound
ways, incarcerated women, including those who are mothers, represent
a neglected population. Their health problems and health care needs
are rarely studied (Ingram-Fogel, 1991). Male inmates receive most of
the programs and services including medical, dental, recreational,
educational, and vocational (Arditi, Goldberg, Hartle, Peters, & Phelps,
1973; Clement, 1993; Goetting, 1985). Moreover, women's programs
and services offered to female inmates are based primarily on models
derived from male inmates (Rafter, 1992); most models for mental
health services in correctional facilities (e.g., Hilkey, 1988) are not

sensitive to gender considerations. As a reflection of society at large, the correctional system responds to women's needs and experiences within the frameworks that represent male perspectives.

The failure to address the needs of incarcerated mothers and other female inmates adequately in a systematic and appropriate way has been justified by prison representatives in the past as well as in the present, based on the fact that women constitute a significantly smaller proportion of the incarcerated population. But the number of women in the correctional system is increasing at an alarming rate (Kline, 1992). For example, between the years 1984 and 1992, the number of women in the federal and state inmate populations went from 20,853 to 50,409 (Bureau of Justice Statistics, 1988, 1991, 1992). In other words, the number of women in prison more than doubled within 8 years.

Women's services should be tailored to meet their needs, because female offenders, including those who are mothers, present a different criminal, psychological, and behavioral profile from their male counterparts. For example, there is a higher proportion of women serving time for nonviolent offenses (i.e., property, drug, and public offenses) as opposed to violent crimes (Bureau of Justice Statistics, 1991).

Not only are the reasons for incarceration different, but the women's psychological profile differs as a result of the accumulated effects of histories of physical, sexual, and emotional abuse; battering; societal marginalization; and an overemphasis on gender-based expectations, such as caretaking and docility. This profile is complicated by the lack of understanding of the actual psychological development process of women, for instance, that described by Jean Baker Miller, Alexandra G. Kaplan, Judith V. Jordan, Irene P. Stiver, and Janet L. Surrey, theorists at the Stone Center, who emphasize the centrality of relationships as the core of psychological life (Jordan, Kaplan, Miller, Stiver, & Surrey, 1991).

Moreover, women's behavioral profiles within correctional institutions are distinct from men's in other respects (Turnbo, 1992). Women more often manifest depression and suicidal thoughts, sexual aggression, nonparticipation and isolation, false bravado/docility, complex physical symptoms, and lack of self-esteem. These presenting problems are further exacerbated by their lower educational attainment, lack of job skills, and sketchy work histories. In short, female inmates present unique characteristics and behavioral profiles that have a profound impact on how women are perceived and managed within correctional institutions.

## DOUBLE JEOPARDY: BEING A WOMAN AND A MOTHER IN PRISON

"I miss them and they miss their mother. It is the hardest thing . . . to be a mother in jail, because I can't be the mother I was raised to be . . . like my mother bring me up."

A majority of women in prison are mothers. Recent statistics show that about 75% of all women in prison are mothers (Bureau of Justice Statistics, 1991). The needs of this particular population, including those of the children and other family members left behind, has just recently begun to be acknowledged (Baunach, 1988; Bloom & Steinhart (1993).

What do we know about these mothers? The media's portrayal of mothers in prison is mixed, ranging from editorials asserting that children would be better off cared for by relatives or in foster families than by their parents in prison (e.g., "Moms in Jail," 1995), to articles advocating programs that allow women to keep their infants in prison settings or increase their access to their children (e.g., Cummings, 1993; Jose-Kampfner, 1992; "Maternal Bonds," 1990; Harris, 1993). Recently, there has been some acknowledgment of the complexity of the situation as more women are incarcerated and thus more children are left behind (Applebome, 1992, 1994).

Many articles highlight advances in correctional institutions as they recognize that learning how to be good parents is a key part of prison rehabilitation (e.g., Verde, 1991; Davis, 1995; DeAngelis, 1995). Although written with an overtone of sympathy, most articles present incarcerated mothers as inadequate, incompetent, and unable to provide adequately for the needs of their children. After all, how can a person with a criminal record be a "good" mother?

The academic literature reflects the same biases against incarcerated mothers. One set of literature emphasizes their inadequacies as parents. The basic argument is that most mothers (and fathers) in prison need to improve their parenting skills (Tilbor, 1993; Ripley, 1993), especially because they have often neglected and abused their children prior to incarceration and will regain custody when released from prison. The assumption is that these parents really do not care about the well-being of their children. In other words, the lack of investment in their parenting role is one of the reasons that they are in prison. They have chosen (so goes the argument) to abandon their children by being in conflict with the law.

A second bias in the academic literature is the emphasis only on the children (and society) as victims, neglecting the idea of the mothers themselves suffering (Bloom & Steinhart, 1993; Barry, 1985; McGowan & Blumenthal, 1978). In this literature, the impact of the mothers' incarceration is viewed as devastating to their children and as having an impact upon many individuals other than the women themselves. Because parental incarceration can have a negative impact on the emotional, behavioral, and psychological development of children (Hairston, 1991), these women's crimes and consequent punishment is presented as that much more devastating to society.

Despite some media and academic acknowledgment that children's needs are unmet and that incarcerated mothers need support in exercising their parenting skills, the biases that permeate the response by the criminal justice system and the public at large to incarcerated mothers result in prison environments that are usually not supportive of parent–child relationships (Bloom & Steinhart, 1993; Johnston, 1995). Although some special programs have been developed and met success in bringing prisoners and their families together (Boudoris, 1995; Moses, 1995), these efforts are scattered.

Further, negative views about incarcerated mothers, unfortunately, are shared by correctional staff. In a study by Henriques (1982), 30% of the institutional personnel interviewed perceived incarcerated mothers as irresponsible, uncaring, and lacking discipline in their mothering role. In addition, 26% viewed them as manipulative and selfish, and another 22% viewed them as immature. The negative views on the part of correctional staff toward these mothers have clear implications for how the women are treated during incarceration.

## THE IMPACT OF INCARCERATION ON MOTHERS THEMSELVES

"I've had contact with him but . . . they won't bring him. They are giving me a hard time about transportation. And my children are the closest thing to me whether they're with me or not . . . and it's so very painful."

Concerned mostly with the children's well-being, very few studies have paid attention to the mothers themselves: How do these women experience motherhood behind bars? How does the separation from their children affect them? How do they conceptualize motherhood?

The few studies that exist suggest that although many incarcerated mothers are not meeting their parental responsibilities, they are keenly aware of what these responsibilities are. Of primary concern is their physical presence. Henriques (1982) reports that 44% of her sample cited that separation from their children was their main concern and that they were deeply affected by it. The mothers' definition of their role was as follows: to provide emotional care and support (60%), teach their children (40%), provide physical care and support (33%), and possess personal attributes (e.g., patience) that lead to better understanding and interaction with their children (33%).

Similarly, Baunach (1985) in the introduction to her seminal study of mothers in prison summarizes the scant research conducted to date and reports the common threads in the findings: Most mothers are living with their children prior to incarceration, and many of the incarcerated mothers are trying to maintain contact with their children and are planning to reunite with them after release. This is the case despite little support from most correctional institutions in maintaining ties between mothers and children during and after incarceration. Similar findings are reported in a more recent study by Bloom and Steinhart (1993).

In spite of these mothers' seemingly important investment in their children, Baunach (1985) comments that the role that inmate mothers play as parents during their incarceration is minimal as a result of the nature of the correctional system. Given these constraints, it is not surprising that mothers express feelings of inadequacy, despondency, and fear of permanent loss of their children. Furthermore, because their own behavior has caused the separation, most mothers feel intense guilt and shame. They also express fears of not being able to regain respect and authority from their children and of being rejected by them. In spite of all these obstacles, based on her research and that of others, Baunach argues that the role of mother appears to be a very central aspect of the lives of these women, a source of self-esteem, self-definition, and identity as a woman.

## DOCUMENTING INCARCERATED MOTHERS' EXPERIENCES

"If I am in jail or not, I can still be a good mother."

Most of the public discourse on incarcerated women, including those who are mothers, does not reflect these women's voices. This chapter, in contrast, will concentrate on presenting the voices of incarcerated mothers extrapolated from two different sources. The first source is a study conducted by the Stone Center for Developmental Services and Studies at Wellesley College in which two of the authors (C.G.C. & J.L.S.) participated. The second source reflects the clinical and administrative experiences of the other authors of this chapter (P.B.-N.& B.M.) and the information they gained by conducting a focus group with incarcerated women. The following describes the two sources in more detail.

The Stone Center study was designed to document the particular needs of incarcerated women and the role of relationships in these women's lives (see García Coll & Duff, 1996, for a description of the study background, methodology, and other findings). As part of the inmates' responses to a variety of questions about their past, present, and future needs, spontaneous remarks about their children and their role as a mother were expressed. The investigators were struck by the saliency of the women's identity as mothers while in prison, confirming Baunach's (1985) observations and conclusions.

The study was conducted in a minimum security prerelease correctional facility for men and women in a northeast state in April and May of 1994. At the time of the study, there were 82 women incarcerated in this facility. The women were housed in two buildings adjacent to the men's facilities.

For the purpose of this chapter, we reviewed the transcripts of 11 different focus groups that were led by bicultural, biracial teams of two leaders. One group was conducted entirely in Spanish; some groups were bilingual English and Spanish. Participating voluntarily in the study were 52 women (out of 82 held at this facility). This group of women shared many characteristics representative of women in prison nationwide (Kline, 1992; Massachusetts Department of Correction, 1992). For example, 76% of these women were incarcerated for the first time, 56% for drug related offenses; 47% were minority (African Americans or Latinas); 60% were single; and 80% were mothers (see García Coll, Miller, Fields, & Matthews, 1997, for a more detailed description of the sample).

The review of the transcripts consisted of several steps. First, we read all the transcripts and noted the references to mothering. We extracted comments from the rest of the discourse and conducted a content analysis of these quotes in terms of a framework of resistance. In other words, we asked how these women maintained a sense of their mothering in spite of being incarcerated. How did their actions, thoughts, and feelings constitute resistance against the ultimate punishment (for some of them) of being separated from and not involved in decisions regarding their children?

The second source of the voices presented in this chapter stems from the work of the other two authors (P.B.-N. & B.M.). Both are staff members of Social Justice for Women (SJW), a nonprofit organization incorporated in Boston in 1986. The agency is dedicated to providing substance-abuse treatment, health education, and prison alternatives to women in conflict with the law. SJW specializes in designing and implementing alternatives to incarceration for women who are pregnant, have children, are at risk of HIV infection, or have AIDS. The agency serves women who are prison-bound, incarcerated, or recently released, ages 18 or older, with most clients being between the ages of 20 and 35. Over 75% of the agency's clients are single mothers. They are largely from urban areas, and have limited education and minimal job skills; most are polysubstance addicted; 50% are Caucasian, 27% African American, 22% Latina.

Some of the quotes in this chapter are from women assigned to a substance abuse treatment recovery unit in the Women in Recovery Program in a house of correction in a northeast state. The unit houses up to 32 women who have histories of substance abuse and who are serving sentences of less than 2.5 years. A focus group was conducted with all women participating, followed by a voluntary survey to which 11 women responded.

Further information presented is based on clinical observations of residents at the Neil J. Houston House (NJHH), a minimum security, community-based prerelease facility for pregnant women with histories of substance-abuse. The facility may house up to 15 women and their infants. Women are within an 18-month-sentence structure. An admission requirement for the NJHH is that the women desire to parent the baby they are carrying, and parenting instruction is an important component of the program. Most of the women also indicate that they wish to be reunited with their other children at some point in the future and look to the program for support and guidance in this area. Both the substance-abuse recovery unit and the NJHH are operated by SJW.

For all of us who have been in contact with these mothers, as researchers and clinicians, the experience has had a profound impact. We have felt along with these women a deep commonality of the female and mothering experience in this society. We realized that the differences between us were mostly in the access to resources throughout our lifetime, but not in our wishes and dreams for ourselves and our families in the present and in the future. As such, getting to know these women has made us realize the privileges in our lives, and we have gained a deeper understanding of their struggles as women and mothers in this society. What we have learned from them is invaluable, though painful and frustrating at times. We hope that by presenting their voices we can share with others the complexity of their situation and life choices.

## SOURCES OF MARGINALIZATION FOR INCARCERATED MOTHERS

Q: Give me an example of what you look forward to as being the sweetest thing about freedom?

A: Taking care of my children.

There are several ways incarcerated mothers are marginalized. The foremost is their definition by the criminal justice system, which identifies them solely as criminals. For that reason, their management within the criminal justice system is guided by the principle that they are here solely to be punished for their crimes. Whatever other negative consequences follow (e.g., separation from young children, losing custody of children, negative consequences to children, etc.) do not concern the criminal justice system. For example, having visitation rights is a reward for good behavior, not an inherent right of their motherhood. Within the criminal justice system (for the most part), by definition, you cannot be both a criminal and a good mother. This is in spite of the fact that these women's criminal behavior is usually quite different from men's, as explained above. Yet their treatment within the correctional facilities follows the pattern of men. As an incarcerated mother states it:

> "The men get in trouble . . . [and so at the prison] they bear down on the women. The women are abiding by the rules . . . we did not go out and shoot a cop . . . they did. We do not escape . . . they do. We wear the proper clothes that we are supposed to . . . they don't. The women will take care of themselves because we want to see our kids. We want to go home. We want to be quiet. I mean you don't have a rowdy bunch of women here."

If per chance incarcerated women's status as mothers becomes relevant, the assumption is that these women have to prove themselves worthy of their motherhood. Incarcerated mothers have to prove competency; they cannot expect support for their mothering role. It is implicitly assumed that by choosing crime, they have chosen to abandon their children.

A similar source of marginalization is the larger society's response to these women's incarceration. In the media, in general, women prisoners are demonized and presented as morally degenerate. These views are not only public representations, but are internalized by the women themselves, their families, and their support systems. Many of these women's families and support systems choose to disconnect with them during and after their prison term. Incarceration brings shame, and the fact of incarceration is often hidden or not acknowledged.

Unlike male prisoners, whose mothers, wives, and girlfriends visit and bring children, it has been our experience that female prisoners are frequently abandoned by those most connected to them. Husbands, boyfriends, and family members often refuse to bring children for a variety of reasons. These reasons include unwillingness to expose children to a prison setting, matters of travel and time, and custody arrangements. As an incarcerated mother expresses it:

"Well, I have seen them once since I have been in . . . and then he [ex-husband] turned around and said, 'Don't think you're ever going to see them again, because you are not.' So it's going to be a long fight. I want to get my kids back."

Some women choose not to exercise their visitation rights, due to the pain of being seen by their children in a prison setting. One mother who has not seen her children since the beginning of her incarceration says, "I feel not to see them because it feels like [it will be] a lot of pain for me as well as for they."

Other sources of marginalization include the consequences of the frequently observed lack of internal resources of incarcerated mothers, resources that could otherwise support their mothering role. This is a result of dysfunctional or deprived family systems that did not allow or support their own healthy growth and development, the resulting psychological consequences of histories of childhood and adult trauma and experiences of violation, and years of substance use and abuse.

These developmental histories can lead to behaviors that further marginalize them: poor educational and employment track records, destructive or immature life choices, and so forth. In describing her family situation, one incarcerated woman states:

> "As far as my family situation . . . if it wasn't sexual abuse it was physical abuse. My sister went through it . . . she is considered mentally slow because of it. My brother has been in jail for all his life because of sexual abuse."

In addition, a possible consequence of such childhood or adult trauma can be posttraumatic stress disorder (PTSD). Symptoms of PTSD include reexperiencing the event, flashbacks, hypervigilance, exaggerated startle responses and/or dissociations, avoidance of stimuli, and numbing (Herman, 1995). These symptoms can persist if PTSD is unrecognized or unattended. Because many incarcerated women are suffering from PTSD, this has profound implications for the mothering role in many of them. These seemingly irrational behaviors can lead to these women being labeled as crazy, unpredictable, or volatile, or as having serious depression due to unexplained reasons. These labels and/or diagnoses can lead to treatments that further pathologize and marginalize these women. Their adequacy or fitness as mothers may be questioned and may lead ultimately to removal or loss of custody of their children. Instead, a clear diagnosis and appropriate treatment for PTSD could be beneficial not only for the mother, and her management in the correctional facility, but also ultimately for her children.

Further, the SJW experience in working with these women has identified the trauma of incarceration as separate and distinct. That is, further psychological damage caused by the incarceration itself has to be addressed before and after release in order for them to resume their mothering responsibilities. Most women "shut down" emotionally in order to survive in a prison environment. Women must be encouraged to discuss this so that they can become more emotionally available for their children. It is very important to establish therapeutic safety so that women can be emotionally present.

In addition, most incarcerated women have long histories of substance use and abuse. The immediate consequence of addiction may be incarceration, but addiction can have a cumulative negative effect on the mothering role, which ultimately leads to a failure to develop a vision of the future or to create a life plan. Because "feeding" the addiction is paramount, the women may neglect their children and their traditional caretaking role. Therefore, they can't fulfill their hopes and dreams to mother as well or better than their own mothers did. For some, drugs might have been used initially as a support in their attempts to function as a mother, but then addiction keeps them from being the mothers they wish to be: This is a tragedy for them, their children, and society. We need to recognize both their good intentions and their bad judgments that led them into this destructive pathway where their relationship with drugs comes at the expense of other, more crucial relationships in their lives, including those with their children.

It has been SJW's experience that once in recovery, women experience the guilt and shame they have about the kind of mothers they actually were, compared to how they wanted to be. As one mother of a 7-year-old daughter tells it:

> "And it only happened a year ago. . . . We've gotten a mother–daughter relationship. I am a mother now. I wasn't before. I took care of their daily needs. But emotionally I wasn't there for them because I wasn't there for myself. It was the worst time. . . . I can't remember her being a baby, walking, you know a toddler. . . . And it's funny because she is not even with me, but I'm a better mother now than I was before."

Despite the many internal and external obstacles that incarcerated mothers face in their role as mothers, it is all the authors' experience and that of others (e.g., Baunach, 1985) that motherhood remains the central focus of their lives. Our collective experience is that incarcerated women are not saying, "I do not care about my children." However the accumulated experiences of trauma, addiction, and marginalization have severely limited their ability to implement their dreams and hopes for themselves and their children. As one incarcerated woman states:

> "I could not raise my kids properly. I mean I love my kids . . . but at that point in time, what's love? You know, it was never given to me . . . so how do you know?"

For some, the only source of hope after incarceration is their children. When asked why women come back to prison after being released, one mother says:

> "Many women that fall [back] into prison have the problem that their children have been taken away. When they go out to the

street, they don't have anything, they have nothing inside. Because they say, 'I don't have my children, what will I do? I'll go back to the drug again. I will go back to prostitution again. And I'll go back to prison again. Why fight? Why fight if I have nothing?' "

## AGAINST ALL ODDS:
## MOTHERING IN PRISON

"No matter how long I'm in jail or that they get adopted or whatever, that's the one thing they can't take away from me because I am their mother."

Mothering in prison has different shapes and expressions in part as a result of the mothers' own emotional needs, the age of the children, the custody arrangements, and the criminal justice institution itself. There are mothers who are involved in their children's daily lives (e.g., making family arrangements, reading to their children daily over the phone, etc.) and/or have regular visitation hours. There are others who against their wishes, have not had contact for years, have lost custody, or do not know the whereabouts of their children. The common experience for all, however, is pain, guilt, grief, and longing for the future.

The experience of incarcerated mothers is very much a function of the correctional facility and its philosophy toward mothers and their children. A range exists going from one extreme of no recognition of the need to support the mothering process to the other extreme that sees this process as integral for both mother and child.

An example from the supportive end of the spectrum is the previously mentioned special facility, the NJHH, a program of SJW. NJHH is a nationally recognized and acclaimed program designed to respond to three critical needs of this population: pregnancy, addiction, and criminality. The program provides gender-specific, holistic, relational approaches that intervene in the chronic, relapsing nature of addiction and recidivism manifested by this population. The women "serve their time" in a small community-based, prerelease facility that permits them to receive pre- and postnatal care, substance abuse treatment, and life-skills education. The program has been operating since 1989 and has facilitated the birth of 105 babies and 20 mother–infant reunifications, allowing mothers and infants to be together during the crucial first months of the infant's development.

At the NJHH, motherhood is central. Even in this extremely supportive environment, given such centrality, the mothers' fear of losing their children is tremendous, for both internal and external reasons. Observations of the clinical staff at NJHH suggest that many of the new mothers will not put their babies down or allow anybody else to handle them. These behaviors can be easily pathologized as reflective of "lack of boundaries" or "primitive narcissism." Yet a shift can be proposed where these behaviors are seen as a reflection of the centrality of motherhood in these women's lives and how the fear of losing the child is overwhelming. Rather than intrapsychic pathology, these behaviors can be reframed as attempts to resist being separated from their children or the fear of ultimately losing them. In fact, at NJHH the shift and reframing occurs by acknowledging the women's fears of separation, exploring the reality of that separation actually happening *in the past,* and reassuring in group and individual discussion that the program has been created so that the separation won't happen.

For many incarcerated women at NJHH existence centers around their dreams and highly idealized hopes for a better life for themselves and their children. As one mother in recovery states it: "I want to be clean and have all my kids with me and live in a house and have a good job and take trips to Disney World."

For others at NJHH who are separated from their previous children their focus with the new baby is to do it *right* this time: to avoid losing custody of this one. They tend their babies carefully. Sometimes they become obsessed. They bathe and dress them too often; they never let them out of their sight—or their arms. Even within the supportive environment provided by NJHH, these mothers' insecurity in their mothering role is clearly evident. They want it so much, and yet so much can get in the way of actualizing their dreams of motherhood.

The unique, intense experience of mothering provided by NJHH compares to a wide range of other mothers' experiences within the criminal justice system, from regular visitation; through irregular visitation, infrequent visitation, and no visitation at all; to loss of custody. For example, within low-security prisons (as opposed to high security), visitation patterns are more regular and frequent. The minimum-security prison where the study conducted by the Stone Center took place is the only correctional facility in that particular state where a trailer for overnight visits with children is used. In spite of that, many mothers had not seen their children in years.

How do these women cope with the physical and emotional separation from their children, given the centrality of motherhood in many of these women's lives? We have observed that some mothers reframe their definition of mothering to allow for the separation and loss. As two mothers in the low-security prison express it:

> "And my children are the closest thing to me whether they are with me or not."

> "Because whether or not they live with me, I can still be a good mother. I know that today. If I'm in jail or not, I can still be a good mother."

Many mothers in prison maintain their sense of motherhood even if they have given up custody or do not have any contact with their children, and never will. Motherhood becomes abstract and symbolic. The relationship keeps going even if it is neither actualized nor reciprocated. They are still the mother of their children, even if they neither see them now nor ever will. The dream, the fantasy is what keeps them going.

> "I have not seen my oldest son in a long time, 4 years. But I write to him every week. You know, he doesn't get them. But one day he will. So at least he knows I never forget. I've always stayed in contact, whether they receive the letters or not. They're there."

This quote is the more poignant given the fact that she has been writing letters for 4 years knowing that her son is not receiving them, that she has lost custody of him, and that he may never receive these letters or have any further contact with her. But resisting this loss and maintaining a sense of herself as a mother is as much for her sake as it is for his, contributing at this point to her well-being.

In some cases the incarcerated mother's negativism, manipulation, and other seemingly "bad" behavior (e.g., resisting rules and regulations, stealing, or getting into fights) are signs of *resistance for survival* (see the Introduction and Chapter 3, on homeless mothers). As a mechanism to respond to oppression, resistance for survival consists of short-term strategies that are usually crisis oriented (Robinson & Ward, 1991). Using this framework, what might look like self-destructive behaviors can be seen as acting-out behavior resulting from grief, a sense of loss, shame, and guilt from the previous lack of adherence to the socially prescribed and personally desired mothering role. As a mother states it, guilt is a dominant feeling in these women's lives:

"Guilt for not being there for them to help them see life isn't that bad. Not being involved in afterschool activities, making excuses where I'm at to certain people."

Yet for others, being free of alcohol and drugs, being "clean," and having time on their hands has given them an opportunity to reflect on their own mistakes around mothering and their past limitations.

"I've learned self-respect. I've learned how to nurture myself. . . . How to talk to my children. How to care for them, you know, their needs, 'cause they're in recovery, and I've helped them tremendously . . . which I'm proud of, that I could do that. I couldn't do that way back, till I got to a certain point in my recovery, because I was very defensive. . . . You know? I like myself, today. I didn't like myself, I was a basket case. I learned how to feel, I didn't know how to feel. It took me a year, 15 months to learn how to even feel, to thaw out from all the numbness of drinking. "

This new awareness contributes to some deep yearning for what they used to have and do not have at the present. The pain that some of these mothers are experiencing is a major part of their punishment.

"I would love to have my son back in my life. I would love to take all his pain away and start all over. I will be a better mother to him. I love my son, and I miss him very much. I miss him coming into my room at night and crawling into my bed and rubbing my head and saying, 'Ma, I love you.' "

This pain and awareness of their past limitations contributes to their recognition that they need to restructure their lives after being released in order to fulfill their mothering obligations.

"I know when I get out there, I'm not going to deal with all the responsibilities I had before. I'm only going to take care of me and my kids. And that I don't have to be a mother to my sister, my brothers, or whatever, and I don't have to be a mother to them because I'm not their mother. They have their own life; let them live it."

How can we translate the hopes, dreams, and even negative behaviors, which we conceptualize as seeds of resistance, into sources of support for these women's growth in their lives and particularly their mothering roles?

## MARGINALIZATION AND RESISTANCE: IMPLICATIONS FOR SERVICE PROVIDERS

"I dream to have a happy house and help with things they [the children] need help with and go to the children's school open house and talk with the teacher and have their father there as help."

As we have said, the obstacles that incarcerated mothers have to face are many, some even insurmountable. Many women bring histories of early and continuing trauma and histories of substance use and addiction that get in the way of their best intentions to be a "good" mother. Yet their dreams and hopes are high. For some, the prison experience has made them realize their mistakes and the possibilities for change in their mothering. How do we promote their mothering skills, maintain their hopes, and yet help them face the realities of their lives?

Working with them solely on their psychological growth is not enough. Teaching them how to reframe, resist, or cope with insurmountable circumstances (e.g., possibility of losing custody, impossibility of finding jobs after having a criminal record, ostracism from relatives and friends) is necessary, but insufficient. Many of them have experienced pervasive poverty and discrimination. Their mistrust of the system is profound and to a certain extent justified. Their life skills do not match the many demands they will face when they get out of prison—when and if they reunite with their children.

What we propose is a wider recognition of the centrality of motherhood in these women's lives as a source of energy for positive growth. Acknowledgment, respect, and support are necessary for women who are maintaining contact with their children against many barriers, or are redefining their mothering role while in prison. The criminal justice system does not recognize the importance of the mothering role of women in conflict with the law, and incarcerated women face almost insurmountable obstacles to mothering. Unfortunately, the need for comprehensive services for incarcerated women and their children is being recognized at the same time that society is implementing tougher crime policies for both male and female inmates. The pervasive view—that building more prisons and giving harsher sentences is an effective response to crime—further denies the reality and plight of incarcerated mothers and their children.

We propose instead that for incarcerated mothers the seeds of resistance—their involvement with their children in spite of many barriers; their idealized hopes, dreams, and even negative behaviors— be recognized and utilized to develop and design prison-based, community-based, and aftercare services that recognize the crucial role of mothering in their lives. At the same time, we have to recognize that the centrality of motherhood in these women's lives doesn't mean that just because they wish to be effective mothers, they automatically are or will be. There are many internal and external obstacles to surmount. But that wish, that dream can lead to growth in their personal lives and in their mothering role.

Instead of solely providing lessons in how to be a "good" mother or creating further obstacles to their mothering, the criminal justice system and the medical, mental health, legal, and social service systems that these women come in contact with should promote opportunities to parent within a supportive community. It has been observed among women who are in drug rehabilitation programs that the wish to be a good parent to her child may increase her motivation to change (Black et al., 1994). Therefore, recognizing the centrality of the mothering role in their lives becomes an integral part of prevention and treatment programs rather than punishment (Lester, Affleck, Boukydis, Freier, & Boris, 1996).

In addition, we believe that viewing many of these women's behaviors as reactions to multiple external and internal sources of marginalization and as expressions of resistance creates a critical shift for those who work with incarcerated mothers. This shift has very profound implications for treatment and services. It recognizes that these seemingly negative or maladaptive behaviors—albeit difficult to deal with—are not solely the manifestations of inner psychopathology. The frustration of dealing with these behaviors can be alleviated by reconceptualizing them as a response to the women's (present or past) situation and an expression of their resistance. Following this reconceptualization, treatment services that are based in solidarity, empathy, and mutuality may lead to very different kinds of behavior change and healing. Allowing women to speak, listening to what is really important to them and providing a relational context that does not patholo- gize, label, or objectify their experience can contribute to therapeutic growth and reduce recidivism. In such a context, we might not see so much resistance for survival as a way of coping with loss. When women feel heard, respected as individuals, and connected with others who care about their well-being, negative behaviors decrease. Until such treatment approaches are institutionalized by those working with incarcerated mothers, supporting the seeds of resistance during and after their prison experiences is critical.

## ACKNOWLEDGMENTS

We want to thank all the women who have so kindly shared their lives, views, and experiences with us. The study conducted at the Stone Center was funded by the Massachusetts Committee on Criminal Justice. Many people were integral part of the conduct and analyses of that study: Kathy Duff, Jean Baker Miller, Jacqueline Fields, Sandra Yarney, Erika Stewart, Julia Perez, Yvonne Jenkins, Margaret Potter, Joey Fox, and Heidie Vázquez García. More recently Jesse Sharkey and Suzie Nacar contributed to this chapter.

## REFERENCES

Applebome, P. (1992, November 30). U.S. prisons challenged by women behind bars. *The New York Times*, Section A, p. 10.

Applebome, P. (1994, December 27). Holding fragile families together when mothers are inmates. *The New York Times*, Section 4, p. 2.

Arditi, R. R., Goldberg, F., Hartle, M. M., Peters, J. H., & Phelps, W. R. (1973). The sexual segregation of American prisons. *Yale Law Journal, 82*(6), 1229–1273.

Barry, E. (1985). Children of prisoners: Punishing the innocent. *Youth Law News*, pp. 12–13.

Baunach, P. J. (1985). *Mothers in prison*. New Brunswick, NJ: Transaction Books.

Black, M. M., Nair, P., Kight, C., Wachtel, R., Roby, P., & Schuler, M. (1994). Parenting and early development among children of drug-abusing women: Effects of home intervention. *Pediatrics, 94,* 440–448.

Bloom, B., & Steinhart, D. (1993). *Why punish the children?: A reappraisal of the children of incarcerated mothers in America.* San Francisco: National Council on Crime and Delinquency.

Boudouris, J. (1985). *Prisons and kids: Programs for inmate parents.* College Park, MD: American Correctional Association.

Bureau of Justice Statistics. (1988). *Sourcebook of criminal justice statistics, 1987.* Washington, DC: U.S. Government Printing Office.

Bureau of Justice Statistics. (1991, March). *Women in prison* [Special report]. Washington, DC: U.S. Government Printing Office.

Bureau of Justice Statistics. (1992, May). *Prisoners in 1991* [Special report]. Washington, DC: U.S. Government Printing Office.

Clement, M. J. (1993). Parenting in prison: A national survey of programs for incarcerated women. *Journal of Offender Rehabilitation, 19*(1/2), 89–100.

Cummings, J. (1993, June 30). Should newborns stay with imprisoned moms? *Atlanta Constitution,* p. A6.

Davis, W. (1995, December 6). Parenting from prison. *The Boston Globe,* p. 91.

DeAngelis, M. E. (1995, October 19). Prison brings together inmate moms, children. *Chicago Tribune,* Evening Edition, p. 8.

García Coll, C. T., & Duff, K. M. (1996). *Reframing the needs of women in prison: A relational and diversity perspective* [Project report]. Wellesley, MA: Stone Center.

García Coll, C. T., Miller, J. B., Fields, J. P., & Mathews, B. (1997). The experiences of women in prison: Implications for services and prevention. *Women and Therapy, 20*(4), 11–28.

Goetting, A. (1985). Racism, sexism, and ageism in the prison community. *Federal Probation, 49,* 10–22.

Hairston, C. F. (1991). Family ties during imprisonment. *Journal of Sociology and Social Welfare, 18*(1), 87–104.

Harris, J. (1993, March 28). The babies of Bedford. *The New York Times Magazine,* Section 6, p. 26.

Henriques, Z. W. (1982). *Imprisoned mothers and their children: A descriptive and analytical study.* New York: University Press of America.

Herman, J. (1995). *Trauma and recovery.* New York: Basic Books.

Hilkey, J. H. (1988). A theoretical model for assessment of delivery of mental health services in the correctional facility. *Psychiatric Annals, 18*(12), 676–679.

Ingram-Fogel, C. (1991). Health problems and needs of incarcerated women. *Journal of Prison and Jail Health, 10*(1), 43–57.

Johnston, D. (1995). Parent–child visits in jails. *Children's Environments, 12*(1), 25–38.

Jordan, J. V., Kaplan, A. G., Miller, J. B., Stiver, I. P., & Surrey, J. L. (1991). *Women's growth in connection: Writings from the Stone Center.* New York: Guilford Press.

Jose-Kampfner, C. (1992, April 15). EMU professor looks at effects on kids with mothers in prison. *Michigan Chronicle,* p. C3.

Kline, S. (1992, Spring). A profile of female offenders in state and federal prisons. *Federal Prisons Journal.*

Lester, B. M., Affleck, P., Boukydis, Z., Freier, K., & Boris, N. (1996). Keeping mothers and their infants together: Barriers and solutions. *New York University Review of Law and Social Change, 22,* 425–440.

Massachusetts Department of Correction. (1992, November 25). *Female of-*

*fenders in Massachusetts: Statistical descriptions, trends, and population projections.* Research Division, Massachusetts Department of Correction.

Maternal bonds behind prison bars. (1990, September 23). *The New York Times,* Section 1, p. 34.

McGowan, B., & Blumenthal, K. (1978). *Why punish the children?: A study of children of women prisoners.* Hackensack, NJ: National Council on Crime and Delinquency.

Moms in jail. (1995, June 16). *Houston Chronicle* [Editorial], p. A46.

Moses, M. C. (1995, October). *Keeping incarcerated mothers and their daughters together: Girl Scouts behind bars.* National Institute of Justice, U.S. Department of Justice.

Rafter, N. H. (1992, Spring). Equality or difference? *Federal Prisons Journal.*

Ripley, P. (1993). *Prison education's role in challenging offending behaviour* (Mendip Papers MP 047). Bristol, UK: Staff College.

Robinson, T., & Ward, J. V. (1991). "A belief in self far greater than anyone's disbelief": Cultivating resistance among African American female adolescents. In C. Gilligan, A. G. Rogers, & D. L. Tolman (Eds.), *Women, girls and psychotherapy: Reframing resistance.* Binghamton, NY: Harrington Park Press.

Tilbor, K. (1993). *Prisoners as parents: Building parenting skills on the inside* (Handbook). Edmund S. Muskie Institute of Public Affairs, University of Southern Maine, Portland.

Turnbo, C. (1992, Spring). Differences that make a difference: Managing a women's correctional institution. *Federal Prisons Journal.*

Verde, T. (1991, April 7). Maine prison program helps inmates be good parents. *Boston Globe,* p. B2.

# Conversation Three

*Edited by*

## KATHY WEINGARTEN

*T H E* previous conversations have pointed out the myriad ways that cultural messages can be internalized and make mothers and their children see that their own way of life, their very way of being, is wrong. This can happen for mothers who are "armed" against devaluing messages and for those who are not. In the conversation that follows, new themes are mentioned. In this conversation, we resist the characterization of the mothers in this book as "bad" as we talk about ways in which these mothers—ourselves—are women of value.

CYNTHIA GARCÍA COLL: There is a prevalent notion that when you become a mother your personal development stops. You become Mother, and your efforts shift totally to encouraging the development of the child. This is a fundamental myth.

BETSY SMITH: I agree. In terms of teen mothers, becoming a mother can be a way of healing one's own psychological development. With adoptive mothers, there are challenges that can be enriching, ones that can move them to a more complex identity.

KATHY WEINGARTEN: I'll mention a commonality between incarcerated moms and welfare moms too. Many of them are in desperate situations, and yet they are able to think of themselves as good mothers.

ELIZABETH SPARKS: There are strategies that women use to maintain their views of themselves as "good" mothers. Welfare moms equate managing to put food on the table and a roof over their children's head with being a good mother. It shifts the focus from some abstract ideal and helps them maintain their sense of being a good mother.

PHOEBE KAZDIN SCHNITZER: I think of the importance of role modeling in being a mother. And yet, we demonize these mothers. The culture says, in effect, how can a welfare mother be a role model? How can a teen mother be a good role model? How can an incarcerated mother be one?

KATHY WEINGARTEN: The culture lacks a belief that these groups have something to offer. But any of these groups of moms, in fact, may have qualities to be admired or emulated.

ELIZABETH SPARKS: Yes, it begs the question about culturally determined definitions of people. These particular groups of mothers are not seen as having or being of value.

PHOEBE KAZDIN SCHNITZER: In terms of development, the global view is that their lives are over. For instance, "welfare" is seen as a situation that is stagnant as well as tainted.

CYNTHIA GARCÍA COLL: In addition to the notion that their lives are over, there is also the idea that a mom who is now 40, but who was a teen mom, still feels the repercussions of that early life event, and will forever. It is as if there is an irreparable shift in the life course. Her life story was set at the time of the teen birth.

KATHY WEINGARTEN: The notion is that the mothers' stories stop, become comingled with or taken over by their children's stories. When this happens for mothers, it limits the stories that their children can tell as well. The stories of their mothers as people are missing for them.

LAURA BENKOV: Both the welfare mothers' and prison mothers' stories occur in a societal context that does not address issues of the working poor. These stories are context specific, but the context is often ignored by others. The shape of the teen mothers' lives is also dependent on context, in much the same way. With prison mothers, the institutional structure makes community much harder, if not impossible, to create. Former inmates are not allowed to congregate; they may not spend time together. Mothers are in prison together, but they cannot stay connected when they leave.

KATHY WEINGARTEN: It's interesting that moms who are 18 to 20 years old are lumped in the category of "teen moms" when they would be considered "old" in other parts of the world. Yet, I believe that the lumping together of the older moms with the younger ones is purposeful, to pad the impression of how many teen moms there are. We need to resist the notion that teen parenting is of epidemic proportions.

JANET L. SURREY: In thinking about resistance, I think about building communities of resistance. Currently, there are psychologically oriented "support" services around adoption. We need other kinds of communities of resistance in which older adoptive moms can be used as resources.

KATHY WEINGARTEN: Teen women do seem to form community with other young women who are having children.

CYNTHIA GARCÍA COLL: Yes, but it is viewed as a "bad scene."

KATHY WEINGARTEN: The young women see each other as a resource, though.

CYNTHIA GARCÍA COLL: Just as the criminal justice system sees former inmates connecting with each other as negative, so too does society view teen moms supporting each other as negative.

KATHY WEINGARTEN: Yes. That is so ironic. Just as the center of their lives shifts from their boyfriends to an appreciation of their women friends, they are demonized again.

JANET L. SURREY: Resistance to the demonizing does take place. There are stories of people who challenge these myths successfully.

CYNTHIA GARCÍA COLL: Women in prison may have the most difficult time in developing resistance strategies. For women who are incarcerated, there are structural barriers that actually prevent mothering. That is the bottom line.

LAURA BENKOV: I agree. Any real concern a system has for children is negated when that system punishes a mother without thinking of the consequences for her children. The criminal justice system does punish children when punishing women. Truthfully, it doesn't pay attention to children's welfare. It is graphic when we discuss women on welfare and women who are incarcerated.

CYNTHIA GARCÍA COLL: Graphic, and it ignores the centrality of mothering in these women's lives. These women yearn to be in relationship with their children and with others.

JANET L. SURREY: You might say that the yearning to be in relationship
to others, particularly other mothers, is the reason for this book.
It is why we have juxtaposed different voices and different stories.
It is why we have wanted to think collectively about how marginalization affects mothers and about their sources of resistance. We
hope that the collection of chapters themselves creates a kind of
community, one that can be a voice for liberation.

## *Index*